Big Data in Otolaryngology

Big Data in Otolaryngology

Edited by

Jennifer A. Villwock, MD

Professor, Otolaryngology-Head and
Neck Surgery, The University of Kansas Medical Center,
Kansas City, KS, United States

ELSEVIER

Publisher: Sarah Barth
Acquisitions Editor: Jessica McCool
Editorial Project Manager: Billie Jean Fernandez
Production Project Manager: Fahmida Sultana
Cover Designer: Christian Bilbow

3251 Riverport Lane
St. Louis, Missouri 63043

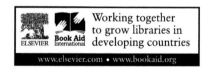

Working together to grow libraries in developing countries

www.elsevier.com • www.bookaid.org

Contents

**CHAPTER 8   The patient perspective on big data and
its use in clinical care 133**

*Katie Tai, MD, Christopher Babu, BS, Medical Student,
Yeo Eun Kim, BS, Medical Student, Tejas Subramanian, BS,
Medical Student and Anaïs Rameau, MD, MPhil, MS, FACS*

Contributors

Kelsey A. Duckett, MD
Department of Otolaryngology-Head and Neck Surgery, Medical University of South Carolina, Charleston, SC, United States

Christopher Babu, BS, Medical Student
Department of Otolarngology - Head and Neck Surgery, New York Presbyterian - Weill Cornell, New York, NY, United States

Andrés M. Bur, MD, FACS, Associate Professor
Department of Otolaryngology—Head and Neck Surgery, University of Kansas, Kansas City, KS, United States

Matthew G. Crowson, MD, MPA, MASc, MBI, FRCSC
Department of Otolaryngology-Head & Neck Surgery, Massachusetts Eye & Ear, Boston, MA, United States

Nathan Farrokhian, MD
Department of Otolaryngology—Head and Neck Surgery, University of Kansas, Kansas City, KS, United States

Elisabeth Ference, MD, MPH, Physician/Surgeon
Division of Otolaryngology, Children's Hospital Los Angeles, Los Angeles, CA, United States

Evan M. Graboyes, MD, MPH
Department of Otolaryngology-Head and Neck Surgery, Medical University of South Carolina, Charleston, SC, United States; Public Health Sciences, Medical University of South Carolina, Charleston, SC, United States

G. Richard Holt, MD, MSEng, MPH, MABE, MSAM, D Bioethics
Professor Emeritus, The University of Texas Health Science Center at San Antonio, San Antonio, TX, United States

Molly P. Jarman, PhD, MPH
Center for Surgery and Public Health, Department of Surgery, Brigham and Women's Hospital, Boston, MA, United States

Rohith (Reddy) Kariveda, BA
Boston University Chobanian and Avedisian School of Medicine, Boston, MA, United States

Yeo Eun Kim, BS, Medical Student
Department of Otolarngology - Head and Neck Surgery, New York Presbyterian - Weill Cornell, New York, NY, United States

Andrew P. Michelson, MD
Department of Pulmonary Critical Care, Washington University School of
Medicine, St. Louis, MO, United States; Institute for Informatics, Data Science &
Biostatistics, Washington University School of Medicine, St. Louis, MO, United
States

Anaïs Rameau, MD, MPhil, MS, FACS
Sean Parker Institute for the Voice, Weill Cornell Medical College, New York, NY,
United States

Nicholas A. Rapoport, BS
School of Medicine, Washington University in St. Louis, St. Louis, MO, United
States

Robert S. Semco, BS
Harvard Medical School, Boston, MA USA

Matthew A. Shew, MD
Department of Otolaryngology-Head and Neck Surgery, Washington University
School of Medicine in St. Louis, St. Louis, MO, United States

Jennifer J. Shin, MD, SM
Department of Otolaryngology - Head and Neck Surgery, Harvard Medical
School, Boston, MA, United States

Tejas Subramanian, BS, Medical Student
Department of Otolarngology - Head and Neck Surgery, New York Presbyterian -
Weill Cornell, New York, NY, United States

Katie Tai, MD
Department of Otolarngology - Head and Neck Surgery, New York Presbyterian -
Weill Cornell, New York, NY, United States

Jennifer A. Villwock, MD
Professor, Otolaryngology-Head and Neck Surgery, The University of Kansas
Medical Center, Kansas City, KS, United States

Big data—Science fiction or clinically relevant?

Matthew G. Crowson, MD, MPA, MASc, MBI, FRCSC

Department of Otolaryngology-Head & Neck Surgery, Massachusetts Eye & Ear, Boston, MA, United States

Introduction

The arrival of cheaper computing power and the proliferation of digital devices, wearables, and innumerable other systems armed with sensors has heralded the "big data" era. The definition of "big data" varies by domain and individual expert opinion. It is commonly accepted to be characterized by data and datasets that are extremely large, such that new techniques and computational approaches are required for processing and analysis.

Today's healthcare systems and their constituents are among the most complicated social, political, and technical structures. This complexity produces immense volumes and a variety of data types. The "big data" generated by nearly every facet of healthcare systems has been of particular interest to stakeholders ranging from patients to clinicians to industry partners (Fig. 1.1). There are many opportunities for harnessing these "big data" to improve healthcare and care delivery. They include fueling the development of artificial intelligence (AI)/machine learning systems from applications as diverse as infectious disease outbreak prediction, novel drug, and device discovery, medical education simulation, clinical trial design, and enhanced diagnosis and prognosis prediction. Other possibilities include using big data to catalyze precision medicine and help solve healthcare delivery challenges such as supply chain and resource procurement.

As the interest in big data in medicine has exploded, so has the enthusiasm in applying "big data" analyses to basic science and translational challenges in *otolaryngology-head and neck surgery*. Over the past 10 years, there has been an exponential rise in peer-reviewed publications relevant to developing AI models using "big data."[1-4] There has been a concomitant surge in interest in leveraging "big data" to produce massive multimodal genetic and omics datasets to push precision medicine forward in fields such as head and neck oncology and otology.[5-8]

This brief chapter aims to provide a brief overview of several current limitations and opportunities for applying big data and AI to *otolaryngology-head and neck surgery*.

Big Data in Otolaryngology. https://doi.org/10.1016/B978-0-443-10520-3.00002-2

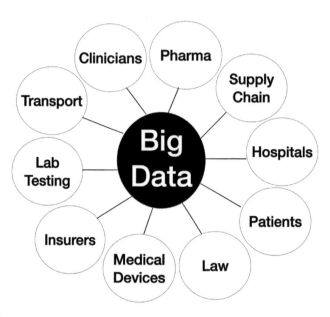

FIGURE 1.1

Big data is involved in all facets of healthcare.

Limitations of big data

The bright future for *otolaryngology-head and neck surgery* in the "big data" era, and the applications for how "big data" may impact the specialty, seem endless. However, we must temper this enthusiasm for the ability of "big data" to transform healthcare by acknowledging several important limitations that must be addressed before the full potential of "big data" in *otolaryngology-head and neck surgery* is realized.

Computational power

In the 1960s, a prominent semiconductor researcher predicted that the number of transistors—a key component of computer chips—would double every 2 years, commensurate with advances in the computer chip manufacturing.[9] This prediction often referred to as "Moore's Law," would serve as a benchmark for predicting the rate of innovation in computing and technology. Remarkably, Moore's law has maintained a reasonable accuracy over time.[10] This observation provides the context for how computing has evolved over the years from bulky, room-filling machines to powerful miniaturized computers found in smartphones everywhere in the world.

Despite this exponential rise in computing power, data generation volume and velocity are—and have—outpaced our analytic and computational capabilities.[11] In 2020 alone, it is estimated that healthcare systems and entities worldwide generated around 2314 exabytes of new data.[12] For context, 1 exabyte is the equivalent of 1 million terabytes—and 2314 exabytes refers to the amount of *new* healthcare data generated in 2020. Considering that today's high-performance computer systems are typically equipped with hard drives of gigabytes or terabytes with read-access memory topping out in the gigabytes, we find that many "big data" analyses are not possible for the average user or research institution. As a result of this constraint, investigators and researchers are forced to handle smaller, less complex datasets on local hardware.

To get around the size of big data in healthcare, some teams are shifting toward cloud computing platforms that promise to offer more computational power without the need to dedicate physical space, upkeep, and capital investment in on-premises hardware. The field of quantum computing is also garnering some interest in applications for extensive data analysis with computational speeds that are orders of magnitude faster than existing computer chip architectures.

Ethical considerations

One of the key benefits of AI is the ability to produce predictions and output at a velocity and scale that no human can replicate. While mass-producing benefit is desirable and improperly designed, AI systems might also disproportionately amplify undesirable outcomes, including bias, privacy violations, and accountability.[13,14]

Fairness and bias

Fairness and bias, in the context of machine learning in healthcare, generally refer to algorithmic output that unfairly favors, or is against, individuals or groups of individuals. Bias may arise at any point in the model development lifecycle, but biased data sources and collection (i.e., ascertainment bias) have been a significant concern. Appraisals of published healthcare AI concepts and deployments have demonstrated bias in data sourcing from discrete geographical locales (e.g., majority United States of America and east Asia), sociodemographic representation (e.g., group underrepresentation related to sex, age, ethnicity, race), and medical specialty representation (e.g., radiology comprising a disproportionate percentage of clinical AI manuscripts).[15] Currently, investigators are developing interventions for various steps in model development pipelines to combat the possibility of biased or otherwise unbalanced datasets and model outputs.

Consent

In contemporary clinical practice, the consent process is integral to patients' autonomy. In the context of the patient–clinician relationship, patients consent to healthcare after a clinician appraises the options, risks, benefits, and expected outcomes of a proposed care plan. Indeed, in the United States, it is a law that clinicians explain medical interventions before they are implemented.[16] However, as we consider where AI algorithms optimally fit into care processes, ethical challenges arise concerning if and how patients should be informed that an AI algorithm is integrated into their care plan.[14] Current medicolegal and regulatory frameworks do not exist for many aspects of healthcare AI implementation, including clinician-to-patient disclosure of AI algorithms in clinical contexts.

Privacy

Healthcare AI models typically require significant volumes of data, and such data may include sensitive information. Privacy preservation for healthcare data is neither new nor unique to AI, but the mass mobilization of data to power AI algorithms underscores the importance of data privacy. Key data privacy issues to consider in the AI model lifecycle include (1) who should and should not access sensitive data; (2) the security of cloud versus on-premises computing environments; (3) secure and effective sharing of data with multiinstitutional or institutional-industry collaborations; (4) safeguarding against adversarial attacks of deployed AI systems that may reveal sensitive features or attributes of the model training data; (5) and the repurposing of existing biomedical data for new models that may differ from the original intent.

Opportunities in big data

As of the writing of the manuscript, big data has powered innovations in virtually every step of the healthcare journey:

- **Evaluation and management** (e.g., "smart" scribes, autonomous triage tools and decision support, high-throughput preventative health measure screening, and risk stratification),
- **Diagnostics** (e.g., AI-augmented radiology software, point-of-care medical devices),
- **Therapies** (e.g., individualized chemotherapy medication assignment based on—omics data, drug discovery),
- **Prognostication** (e.g., intervention outcomes prediction using multimodal data, enhanced modeling of complex clinicopathologic relationships), and
- **Healthcare systems operations** (e.g., supply-chain modeling and automated procurement, "Black Swan" event prediction and crisis scenario modeling, public health program monitoring and prediction)

The opportunities for big data to innovate and advance healthcare delivery in *otolaryngology-head and neck surgery*, as outlined above, are exciting and within grasp.

Capturing interconnectedness using graph data and network analysis

Graph data are comprised of nodes and edges representing relationships between defined nodes (Fig. 1.2). Graph data can be used to model and understand complex

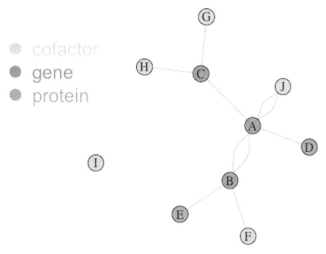

FIGURE 1.2

Example graph depicting connections (i.e., the links) between genes, proteins, and cofactors (i.e., the nodes)—sample data and code generated in R with the *igraph* package.

relationships between virtually any type of discrete biomedical entity, such as genes, proteins, patients, symptoms, drugs, surgeries, or other events. Links between such entities can be measured and defined according to directionality or the strength of association. The field of network analysis aims to use graph data as a medium for analytical tasks such as cluster identification, relationship prediction, node prediction, and other applications.

To date, relatively little network analysis work has been published in *Otolaryngology-Head and Neck Surgery*. However, network analysis is an emerging area of research and operational interest in healthcare. Graph data approaches have been applied to model chronic disease progression,[17] healthcare fraud risk estimation,[18] infectious disease source identification,[19] and graphical representations of electronic medical record data.[20]

Integrating multimodal data for precision medicine

Precision medicine is a relatively new approach to healthcare delivery whereby care plans are individually tailored to an individual based on their genetic information, environmental contexts, and other factors. The goal of precision medicine is to "target the right treatments to the right patients at the right time."[21] Precision medicine has been made possible through advances in genomic sequencing techniques and a marked decrease in sequencing costs. As of the writing of this manuscript, commercial vendors are offering whole-genome sequencing for individuals at $250–500 USD. The cost of individual whole-genome sequencing was $100,000+ USD just a decade ago.

While precision medicine as it relates to *otolaryngology-head and neck surgery* remains in a nascent stage, the applicability of genomic-based analyses is a natural fit for disciplines such as head and neck oncology. Early scoping reviews have identified differential prognosis and targeted therapeutic pathways based on the accumulated knowledge of chromosomal copy number alterations, mutations, and gene expression relevant to head and neck squamous cell carcinoma (HNSCC).[8] Similarly, neurobiological conditions such as tinnitus have also been highlighted as targets for precision medicine given a combination of central and peripheral functional correlates and a rich set of multimodal testing (e.g., traditional audiometry, emissions testing, electromyography, patient-reported outcomes).[7]

Looking ahead

We have only just realized the opportunities for "big data" to advance healthcare and healthcare delivery in *otolaryngology-head and neck surgery*. The healthcare systems in which otolaryngologists work produce immense volumes and a variety of data. Machine learning as a toolkit for big data is more available than ever, and the barriers to entry to developing practical algorithms are low. We are learning how to use network analysis to represent complex relationships better to capture the association between health determinants and disease. Cheaper genomic sequencing will enable investigators to readily incorporate individuals' genomes in research and point-of-care tools for individualized care plans. The opportunities briefly reviewed in this chapter are but a mere glimpse of what is to come.

In addition to the limitations listed herein, some significant constraints and concerns will have to be addressed to unleash the transformative capabilities of "big data." Concerning safeguarding against the ethical problems inherent to the use of AI in healthcare, thoughtful design and deployment of models is prudent. Expressly, concerted efforts to prevent ethical breaches should incorporate governance frameworks for oversight, data, algorithm privacy impact assessments, accessible audit systems, and postdeployment monitoring.[22]

References

1. Bur AM, Shew M, New J. Artificial intelligence for the otolaryngologist: a state of the art review. *Otolaryngol Head Neck Surg.* 2019;160(4):603−611. https://doi.org/10.1177/0194599819827507.
2. Crowson MG, Ranisau J, Eskander A, et al. A contemporary review of machine learning in otolaryngology-head and neck surgery. *Laryngoscope.* 2020;130(1):45−51. https://doi.org/10.1002/lary.27850.
3. Tama BA, Kim DH, Kim G, Kim SW, Lee S. Recent advances in the application of artificial intelligence in otorhinolaryngology-head and neck surgery. *Clin Exp Otorhinolaryngol.* 2020;13(4):326−339. https://doi.org/10.21053/ceo.2020.00654.

4. Wilson BS, Tucci DL, Moses DA, et al. Harnessing the power of artificial intelligence in otolaryngology and the communication sciences. *J Assoc Res Otolaryngol.* 2022;23(3): 319−349. https://doi.org/10.1007/s10162-022-00846-2.

5. Cavalieri S, De Cecco L, Brakenhoff RH, et al. Development of a multiomics database for personalized prognostic forecasting in head and neck cancer: the big data to decide EU project. *Head Neck.* 2021;43(2):601−612. https://doi.org/10.1002/hed.26515.

6. Orlandi E, Licitra L. Personalized medicine and the contradictions and limits of first-generation deescalation trials in patients with human papillomavirus-positive oropharyngeal cancer. *JAMA Otolaryngol Head Neck Surg.* 2018;144(2):99−100. https://doi.org/10.1001/jamaoto.2017.2308.

7. Tzounopoulos T, Balaban C, Zitelli L, Palmer C. Towards a mechanistic-driven precision medicine approach for tinnitus. *J Assoc Res Otolaryngol.* 2019;20(2):115−131. https://doi.org/10.1007/s10162-018-00709-9.

8. Van Waes C, Musbahi O. Genomics and advances towards precision medicine for head and neck squamous cell carcinoma. *Laryngoscope Investig Otolaryngol.* 2017;2(5): 310−319. https://doi.org/10.1002/lio2.86.

9. Schaller RR. Moore's law: past, present and future. *IEEE Spectrum.* 1997;34(6):52−59. https://doi.org/10.1109/6.591665.

10. Edwards C. Moore's law: what comes next? *Commun ACM.* 2021;64(2):12−14. https://cacm.acm.org/magazines/2021/2/250070-moores-law-what-comes-next/abstract.

11. Dinov ID. Volume and value of big healthcare data. *J Med Stat Inform.* 2016;4. https://doi.org/10.7243/2053-7662-4-3.

12. Culbertson N. *The Skyrocketing Volume of Healthcare Data Makes Privacy Imperative.* Forbes; August 6, 2021. Retrieved October 31 from https://www.forbes.com/sites/forbestechcouncil/2021/08/06/the-skyrocketing-volume-of-healthcare-data-makes-privacy-imperative/?sh=277a5a4b6555.

13. (WHO), W. H. O. *Ethics and Governance of Artificial Intelligence for Health.* World Health Organization (WHO); June 28, 2021. Retrieved October 31 from https://www.who.int/publications/i/item/9789240029200.

14. Gerke S, Minssen T, Cohen G. Ethical and legal challenges of artificial intelligence-driven healthcare. In: *Artificial Intelligence in Healthcare.* 2020:295−336. https://doi.org/10.1016/b978-0-12-818438-7.00012-5.

15. Celi LA, Cellini J, Charpignon M-L, et al. Sources of bias in artificial intelligence that perpetuate healthcare disparities—a global review. *PLOS Digit Health.* 2022;1(3): e0000022. https://doi.org/10.1371/journal.pdig.0000022.

16. Astromskė K, Peičius E, Astromskis P. Ethical and legal challenges of informed consent applying artificial intelligence in medical diagnostic consultations. *AI Soc.* 2021;36(2): 509−520. https://doi.org/10.1007/s00146-020-01008-9.

17. Khan A, Uddin MS, Srinivasan U. Adapting graph theory and social network measures on healthcare data: a new framework to understand chronic disease progression. In: *Proceedings of the Australasian Computer Science Week Multiconference.* 2016.

18. Branting LK, Reeder F, Gold J, Champney T. Graph analytics for healthcare fraud risk estimation. In: *2016 IEEE/ACM International Conference on Advances in Social Networks Analysis and Mining (ASONAM).* August 18−21, 2016.

19. Li L, Zhou J, Jiang Y, Huang B. Propagation source identification of infectious diseases with graph convolutional networks. *J Biomed Inform.* 2021;116:103720. https://doi.org/10.1016/j.jbi.2021.103720.

20. Calzoni L, Clermont G, Cooper GF, Visweswaran S, Hochheiser H. Graphical presentations of clinical data in a learning electronic medical record. *Appl Clin Inform*. 2020; 11(4):680−691. https://doi.org/10.1055/s-0040-1709707.
21. (FDA), F. D. A. *Precision Medicine*; September 27, 2018. Retrieved October 31 from https://www.fda.gov/medical-devices/in-vitro-diagnostics/precision-medicine.
22. Bartoletti I. *AI in Healthcare: Ethical and Privacy Challenges*. AIME; 2019.

Large administrative datasets: Lessons and limitations

2

Elisabeth Ference, MD, MPH, Physician/Surgeon

Division of Otolaryngology, Children's Hospital Los Angeles, Los Angeles, CA, United States

Introduction

There is a growing interest in the use of large datasets in otolaryngology research. From 2005 to 2016, there was nearly a 10-fold increase in database publications in major otolaryngology journals.[1] Because these databases contain information for a large patient population, they provide the advantage of having strong statistical power and generalizability, making them an appealing source for observational research with numerous applications. Database studies have made significant contributions to advancing the otolaryngology field. For example, they have facilitated the creation of the AJCC staging systems for multiple cancers.[2] One of the most cited papers in otolaryngology literature utilized a national cancer database to examine the trends in the management of advanced laryngeal cancer.[3,4]

Many large databases derive from hospital administrative data, which are routinely collected for all patients during hospital and clinic visits. Although these datasets were initially designed for healthcare services reimbursements, they are increasingly being used for epidemiological and outcomes research. Critical appraisal of studies that utilize large database is important because there can be inherent problems with the data collection and quality of data that may introduce confounding and biases.

In this chapter, we will first review the overall advantages and limitations of using large databases for research. We will then delve into more detail regarding several common databases that have been used in otolaryngology research, including their individual strengths, weaknesses, and important considerations when choosing each database.

Overview of large databases

Large-volume national databases can be broadly categorized as administrative or clinical registry depending on where the data derive.[5] Administrative databases are compiled from billing information and are not originally intended for clinical research. They obtain their information typically from requests to insurers for

Big Data in Otolaryngology. https://doi.org/10.1016/B978-0-443-10520-3.00008-3

healthcare payments and claims for services. They may be national, state-based, or limited to a specific geographic region. Administrative datasets utilize the *International Classification of Disease* (ICD) codes for diagnoses and *Current Procedural Terminology* (CPT) codes for procedures, relying on coders to interpret the medical records with accuracy. Clinical databases, on the other hand, are developed specifically for clinical care purposes. They are composed from the patient population, with information derived from the patient medical records. These databases are designed to record and track patient information longitudinally, allowing for patient-level investigation of specific clinical questions.

There are two major types of cancer registries: population-based and hospital-based. Based on how they collect data, they offer different perspectives on the United States cancer population. Population-based registries, such as the Surveillance, Epidemiology, and End Results Program (SEER), record all cancer cases in a defined population. These registries are designed to determine the distribution of cancer cases among a certain population and to monitor cancer trends over time. These registries were created to advance the field of cancer prevention and screening, healthcare disparities, and public health interventions to reduce the overall cancer burden in our population. Hospital-based registries, such as the National Cancer Database (NCDB), maintain data on patients who are diagnosed with or treated for cancer in specific healthcare facilities. Data from these registries are collected for the purpose of improving quality of care. The first cancer registry in the United States, the Yale-New Haven Hospital Cancer Registry, was a hospital-based registry.

Strengths of large databases

Administrative datasets provide readily available healthcare data on a large population of patients. This population of patients is typically pooled from multiple hospitals across different geographic regions in the United States, so the results are more nationally representative and generalizable than a single institution study. These datasets can be used to describe national treatment trends, costs associated with healthcare delivery, and temporal trends of diseases.[1] Accessing data from across the country also allows comparisons of healthcare utilization, outcomes, and practice habits by geographic region, which is extremely important to improve the quality of healthcare on an institutional and national level.[6] Large databases with adequate power are especially valuable to study diseases that have low incidences which would make individual studies impractical, as well as research questions that are not feasible for randomized controlled trials. These datasets are typically available publicly to download, although there are some costs and restrictions associated with the use of certain databases.

Limitations of large databases

One inherent limitation of administrative data is related to the motivation behind their formation. Because they were intended for financial and administrative purposes, rather than for the goal of research, they may vary in the criteria for data collection.[6] For example, a common limitation shared by many of these databases is that they are dependent on ICD and/or CPT coding to isolate comorbidities, diagnoses, procedures, and complications. These codes were originally used for billing purposes, and so there may be underreporting of certain diagnoses, procedures, or complications if financially disincentivized.[6]

Data accuracy is also another concerning pitfall of administrative dataset. Coding specialists may not be adequately trained in how to interpret complex medical terms from physician records, which may result in misclassification of diagnoses.[7] Inaccuracy in data tabulation can also be impacted by clinician underreporting, poor documentation, and limitations of the codes themselves. A study investigated how frequently spinal fusion patients were given a diagnosis of anemia with ICD-9 code when their preoperative laboratory work showed a low hematocrit; 14.2% of their patients were considered anemic by hematocrit definition, but only 3.8% were documented as anemic with ICD-9 code.[8] This may suggest that databases are better used for recording straightforward information that is less prone to subjectivity by the coders.

Missing data is another unavoidable issue, which can produce bias and compromise the quality of the results. In addition, administrative datasets typically lack the clinical granularity that is otherwise present in patient medical records.[9] For example, patient-level clinical information may not always be available, such as tumor characteristics, pathology reports, and preoperative diagnostics. Specifics of surgeries, such as intraoperative findings, are also usually not recorded in detail. While data on survival are frequently present, there may not be information on functional morbidity and quality of life measures.

With regards to data analytics, it is important to recognize that various sampling strategies across different databases may lead to inconsistent results even for similar patient cohorts.[10] This is because data can be sampled at a visit-, patient-, or hospital-level, which can introduce sampling bias. Databases that employ a complex sampling design require sampling weights to produce national estimates in order to account for clustering of hospitals, sampling bias, and changes in sampling over time. Even when using a single database, the same hypothesis tested on a slightly different case selection can also lead to disparate results.[11] This proves the need for researchers to provide clear and transparent methodology so that the results are reproducible.

Choosing an appropriate data source begins with carefully assessing the strengths and limitations of each dataset. Several major questions that we think should be considered before selecting a database:

- Does the database rely on accurate sampling on geographics units (e.g., states, healthcare facilities, individual healthcare providers)?
- Is the database only interested in diseases treated in the hospital setting?
- Does the database include only individual hospital records, without linkages to follow specific patients over time?
- Does the database account for the sampling design using weights?
- Does the database have significant changes in data structure or variables collected over time?
- How much does the data cost?
- Can the research question be answered given the limitations of the dataset?

National databases

Administrative dataset

National inpatient sample

The National Inpatient Sample (NIS) is one of the several databases that were developed for Healthcare Cost and Utilization Project (HCUP) funded by the Agency for Healthcare Research and Quality (AHRQ). Compiled annually since 1988, the NIS is the largest all-payer inpatient care database in the United States, capturing approximately five to eight million patients per year. Initially, the NIS included 100% of the discharges from sampling of 20% of the hospitals. It was redesigned in 2012 to represent a stratified sample of 20% of all discharges from hospitals across the nation.[12] The NIS is constructed using a complex sampling design, and obtaining national estimates requires accounting for clustering at hospitals and changes in sampling over time.

The NIS contains hospital stay data that includes patient demographics, diagnoses, procedures, disposition, and length of stay. Each record represents a unique hospitalization and does not identify individual patients, meaning that recurrent hospitalizations for a single patient appear as distinct observations. Researchers should not perform hospital-, state-, and provider-level assessments using NIS. Hospital identifiers are not available, and sampling does not account for uniform representation of all the hospitals. US states are also not a part of the sampling design, thus the discharges recorded from a given state are not representative of all discharges from that state.[9] Similarly, provider-level characteristics are difficult to analyze since the provider code in NIS does not link to a specific procedure and is not reported consistently. The NIS only records inpatient events and does not allow for longitudinal tracking of patients. It does not capture outpatient encounters or observation-only stays, so procedures that are performed in multiple different care settings may be underestimated. When conducting studies investigating nationwide trends, appropriate sampling weights that are provided by HCUP need to be applied to account for the complex sampling design.[13]

Although NIS publications are frequently cited in otolaryngology literature,[1,14] these studies need to be interpreted with caution. In a study that evaluated 120 published studies using data from the NIS, the authors found that 85% of the studies did not adhere to the practices and methodology recommended by the AHRQ for the design and conduct of research.[15] More specifically in otolaryngology literature, 94% of the publications from 2014 to 2017 did not adhere to one or more of the practice guidelines.[15] The authors found that most studies did not actually account for the complex sampling design and therefore did not address the effects of sampling error, clustering, and stratification of data in their methodology. The majority of the studies (80%) also did not acknowledge the changes in the data structure of the NIS over time when analyzing temporal trends for certain diseases. Researchers have also misinterpreted the NIS records as patient-level rather than hospital stay, thus leading to inaccurate prevalence estimates. Understanding the appropriate applications and using the correct methodology to interpret NIS data is necessary to generate sound conclusions.

Clinical registry dataset
National surgical quality improvement program

The National Surgical Quality Improvement Program (NSQIP) database was first conceptualized in 1986 when the Congress mandated that the Veterans Administration (VA) system report its risk-adjusted surgical outcomes. Thereafter, there was a decline in postoperative morbidity and mortality in the VA system.[16] In 2004, the American College of Surgeon (ACS) NSQIP was created to measure and report risk-adjusted surgical outcomes for hospitals across the nation.[17] Since its conception, the ACS NSQIP has spread to nearly 700 hospitals, capturing more than one million surgical cases annually. Unlike NIS, participation in the NSQIP is completely voluntary. There is an annual fee associated with hospital participation and this fee covers all program management and data collection by trained clinical reviewers. Participating hospitals are provided with biannual, risk-adjusted, and case mix-adjusted information to benchmark their surgical outcomes and complication rates with a national mean. The NSQIP Pediatric (NSQIP-P) program was piloted in 2008 to address the surgical outcomes for the pediatric population. The NSQIP-P now includes more than 100 sites and captures more than 150,000 pediatric cases annually. Between 2006 and 2010, 47 otolaryngology departments were contributing data to the program.[18]

NSQIP data are collected by trained surgical clinical reviewers from patient medical records, not from insurance claims. The clinical reviewer randomly selects 40 surgical cases over an 8-day period by a specific formula defined by a protocol.[18] Demographic and socioeconomic information, medical comorbidities, preoperative data including laboratory values, procedures, and certain treatment details are all collected. The database also records a wide range of surgery-specific variables such as operative time, blood transfusion, anesthesia type, and estimated blood loss. It does not contain hospital or clinician identifiers, so variations among specific clinicians cannot be examined. Most outcomes in the NSQIP data are limited to a 30-day follow-up period, including perioperative complications and mortality.[19] For readmissions data, NSQIP captures readmissions that occur within 30 days from surgery, not from discharge. This creates immortal bias where patients cannot be readmitted if they have not been discharged; thus, while they are in the hospital, they are considered "immortal" for this outcome.[20] As a result, NSQIP tends to underestimate readmission rates.

Articles that used NSQIP have examined such topics as 30-day adverse outcomes of pediatric patients undergoing thyroidectomy and comparisons in free tissue transfer outcomes between otolaryngology and other specialties.[21,22] Limitations to the utilization of NSQIP for otolaryngology research pertain to the fact that it is primarily a general surgery database. For the years 2009–12, although 1.2 million cases were captured, only 2% were coded as otolaryngology primary.[23] There are more complication data available in the NSQIP dataset than in other large data sources.[24] However, a few studies have questioned the accuracy of the NSQIP surgical risk calculator to predict outcomes after head and neck surgery.[25] This poor predictive value is likely because factors that are unique to head and neck surgery and microvascular surgery, such as tumor location and stage, history of radiation and chemotherapy, nutritional status, and concomitant tracheostomy, are not accounted for in the database.[26] Lastly, because there is a cost associated with participation, teaching hospitals, academic institutions, and hospitals with higher case volume are disproportionally represented in NSQIP.[27] Only institutions who participate in NSQIP are granted access to the data for research purposes.

National cancer database

The NCDB is a hospital-based clinical cancer registry established in 1989 that collects data from more than 1500 hospitals in the United States selected based on Committee on Cancer (CoC) accreditation. The NCDB covers approximately 30% of the hospitals in the United States but captures more than 70% of all newly diagnosed cancers, making the NCDB the largest clinical cancer registry in the world. The number and density of CoC-accredited hospitals vary throughout the United States as CoC-accredited hospitals tend to be in more urban locations and are larger.[28]

The NCDB shared files are site-specific, meaning that there is a separate PUF for cancers of the head and neck. The database contains more than 80 de-identified variables describing sociodemographic, disease, cancer staging, first course of treatment, adjuvant therapy, complications, and outcomes. Data for overall survival are available, but since NCDB does not collect cause of death, disease-free survival cannot be calculated. Functional outcomes and patient-reported outcomes are not available in the database. NCDB only captures readmissions to the reporting facility.

NCDB has multiple advantages that have made it useful for large-scale cancer research. A specific strength of NCDB is the availability and quantity of treatment data.[29] There are more data on types and timing of treatment available through NCDB than the SEER database. A weakness of NCDB is that variables for socioeconomic status are inferred from zip-code level census data and then collapsed into quartiles.[30] The data therefore lack sufficient granularity to precisely analyze how individual-level differences in income or education level impact treatment and survival outcomes. NCDB requires an application for data and releases specific requested data fields to successful applicants.

Surveillance, epidemiology, and end results program

The SEER program was established in 1975 by the National Cancer Institute (NCI). This population-based registry pools data from several cancer registries based on different geographic regions covering 28% of the US population, capturing approximately a quarter of newly diagnosed cancer cases. These geographic regions are strategically chosen to be representative of the US population. Cancer data collection by a registry begins by identifying people with cancer who have been diagnosed or received medical care in various settings including hospitals, outpatient clinics, radiology departments, laboratories, and surgical centers. These facilities then report new cancer cases to a central cancer registry. The most important distinction between the NCDB and SEER is the perspective that each offers on the US cancer population; NCDB is hospital-based, whereas SEER is population-based.

SEER collects data on patient demographics, clinical information, tumor characteristics, stage of disease, first course of treatment, and patient's vital status. Given its easy accessibility, publications using SEER have been on a rise in the past few decades now with nearly 200 per year.[28] SEER data can be used to answer important epidemiological questions such as the incidence and prevalence of cancer, diagnosis and survival by demographics or stage, and overall and disease-free survival. In otolaryngology, SEER has been used to study a broad range of head and neck cancers from human papillomavirus-positive oropharyngeal squamous cell carcinoma to rare tumors including rhabdomyosarcoma and sarcomas of the paranasal sinuses.[31–33]

SEER data must be interpreted carefully. SEER does not account for migration of patients between registries, so duplicate patient records cannot be distinguished. It is also important to note that the SEER population tends to be more urban, includes more cases from the Pacific region, and has a higher proportion of Asian patients.[34] There is also an important limitation with adjuvant treatment data including radiation therapy and chemotherapy.[35] Several analyses that compared SEER registries to Medicare claims data or medical records review demonstrated that SEER captured fewer adjuvant therapy data. One publication that compared SEER with SEER-Medicare data found that the overall sensitivity was 80% for SEER radiation therapy data and 68% for SEER chemotherapy data.[36] For the variables of radiation and chemotherapy, "no treatment" and "unknown" are grouped together as they cannot be accurately distinguished. There are also potential biases associated with those who received treatment that are not captured in the registry data.[37] Taken together, analyses to compare outcomes conditioned on treatment modality cannot be supported by SEER data.

A direct comparison between SEER and NCDB was performed by a study for subsites of head and neck cancers.[34] They found that although the NCDB and SEER sample cancer cases differently, they were quite similar in terms of the demographic, oncologic, and treatment data. The decision to use the SEER or NCDB should therefore be based on if the variables of interest are available. For example, disease-free survival is only recorded by the SEER database, while overall survival can be found in both the SEER and NCDB. Data for length of stay and readmission within 30 days of surgery are available in the NCDB only. The NCDB provides information regarding severity of patient comorbidity via the Charlson comorbidity score, while the SEER database does not offer detailed comorbidity data. Furthermore, the AJCC staging information is separated into clinical and pathological staging variables in the NCDB while collapsed into one variable in the SEER database.

SEER-medicare

The SEER-Medicare dataset was created from the linkage of the SEER database to Medicare claims. The linkage was first completed in 1991 and has subsequently been updated every 2 years. The Medicare dataset contains additional diagnostic and billing codes for services covered by Medicare including diagnostic tests, procedures, hospice care, and prescription drugs. This database primarily includes patients ages 65 or older. Claims data provide more granular comorbidity data based on ICD coding, and treatment-related information and complications. Use of this SEER-Medicare dataset can also be valuable in certain health disparity studies that wish to remove the effect of insurance on health outcomes, as all the patients in this dataset have the same insurance type. A drawback of this dataset beyond those associated with SEER would be that the generalizability to patients under the age of 65 is highly limited. Because personal identifiers were once used to link SEER to the Medicare data, there is a risk for reidentification although the identifiers have been removed from the SEER-Medicare data. Therefore, the SEER-Medicare data are not public use data files. Investigators are required to obtain approval for specific research questions in order to obtain the data.

Survey dataset
National health and nutrition examination survey
The National Health and Nutrition Examination Survey (NHANES) is a national survey designed to assess the health and nutritional status of adults and children in the United States. First developed in 1960, the NHANES is a program of the National Center for Health Statistics (NCHS), which is a part of the Centers for Disease Control and Prevention (CDC). Since 1999, the program has randomly selected participants from 15 different counties across the country each year, including approximately 5000 people annually. The survey is administered in mobile examination centers, and combines both interviews and physical exams. Each cross-sectional

study cycle in NHANES uses a stratified, multistage probability sampling design with selective oversampling of older people, low-income individuals, and racial minorities to produce nationally representative estimates. For example, during the 1999−2006 cycle, non-Hispanic blacks, Mexican Americans, low-income whites, adolescents aged 12−19 years, and persons older than 60 years were oversampled.[38] During the 2007−10 cycle, Hispanics, non-Hispanic blacks, low-income whites, and persons older than 80 years were oversampled.[39] In more recent surveys for 2011−14 and 2015−18, there was oversampling of Asian Americans.[40] The examination response rates in NHANES generally vary from 60% to 80%.[41]

The NHANES collects data on demographic, socioeconomic, lifestyle, environmental exposure, and medical history. Because of its complex sampling design with differential probabilities of selection and response, appropriate sampling weights must be applied to obtain nationally representative estimates. Multiple studies in otolaryngology have used the NHANES to examine the prevalence, risk factors, and disparities for such topics as hearing loss, oral health, and olfaction.[42−45] While some variables, such as eustachian tube dysfunction and hearing loss, can be measured objectively using tympanometry and audiometry respectively, other variables, such as hearing related behaviors like noise exposure and hearing protection, are based on self-reported history.[43,44] The main limitation to using NHANES data is that many of the questions are subject to recall and reporting bias, and lack controlled objective measures and in-depth information.[46] There is evidence also that survey participants tend to underreport information such as healthcare use.[47] Another source of inaccuracy is misclassification bias associated with certain variables. For example, one of the questions in the NHANES smoking-cigarette use questionnaire classify respondents with a lifetime consumption of <100 cigarettes as "never smokers" and those with >100 as "ever smokers."[48] Despite these limitations, data from NHANES are extremely invaluable and can be used in epidemiological studies to guide the development of public health policy to reduce the burden of otolaryngologic diseases.

National ambulatory medical care survey/National hospital ambulatory medical care survey

The National Ambulatory Medical Care Survey (NAMCS) was established in 1973 to study ambulatory visits to nonfederally employed office-based physicians. The National Hospital Ambulatory Medical Care Survey (NHAMCS) was developed in 1976, and began collecting data in 1992 on the utilization of ambulatory care services in hospital emergency and outpatient departments. The scope of the NHAMCS expanded to include hospital-based ambulatory surgery centers in 2009 and ambulatory surgical centers in 2010. With these modifications over time, the NHAMCS is now comprised three components: hospital outpatient departments, hospital emergency departments, and hospital-based ambulatory surgery locations. It excludes federal, military, and veteran facilities. These cross-sectional surveys are administered annually by the Center for Disease Control's National Center for Health Statistics.

Both the NAMCS and NHAMCS utilize a multistate probability sampling design with physician visit as the sampling unit. NAMCS selects visits using a 3-stage probability sampling design, with sampling of geographic regions, physicians, and visits. NHAMCS uses a 4-stage probability sampling design, with sampling of geographic regions, hospitals, outpatient department clinics, and emergency service areas, and visits.[49] Data will need to be weighted from the complex survey design to produce national estimates.

The databases include data elements for patient demographic characteristics, medical conditions, diagnostic and therapeutic services provided, including medications prescribed. The program recommends that estimates be based on >30 affected observations for a diagnosis of interest with a standard error < 30% of the point estimate to support numeric reliability.[50] Only if these standards are met can estimates be generated to represent all ambulatory care visits in the United States. If these standards are not met, then the data are not considered reliable to represent national trends. Moreover, if < 30 observations are available, then the data should not be published as there is a risk of reidentification.

The strength of NAMCS/NHAMCS is that it provides unique insight into ambulatory care. There are some measures that are not available in other data sources, such as specific visit characteristics and provider/setting characteristics. However, the use of these databases also has some limitations as there are limited clinical variables, disease severity, laboratory measures, and outcome measures. For example, the surveys only allows for five diagnoses, and do not collect information about medication dose and quantity.[50] Nevertheless, the NAMCS/NHAMCS has been used in the otolaryngology literature to examine important topics regarding outpatient care practices and trends, utilization of ambulatory and hospitals visits for specific diseases, and treatment patterns including medications and nonmedications.[51,52]

Pediatric databases

Kid's inpatient database

The Kid's Inpatient Database (KID) was developed in 1997 as part of the family of databases under HCUP. As its name suggests, KID is a publicly available database of pediatric inpatient care that is based on administrative data. It represents a sample of pediatric discharges, ranging from birth to 21 years of age, from all community hospitals in states participating in HCUP. It is the largest pediatric all-payer inpatient care database in the United States, including two to three million discharges per year from 2500 to 4100 hospitals. Because it is based on hospital encounters, the database is not longitudinal and cannot be used to track patients over time.[53] Data are nationally representative, and national estimates can be generated with the application of discharge sampling weights in order to project discharges in KID to discharges from all US community hospitals.

KID database provides a unique perspective to study the inpatient pediatric otolaryngologic population.[54,55] The large sample size of the KID enables examination of rare conditions such as congenital anomalies and uncommon surgeries such as airway reconstruction.[56] The ability of this database to link charges to ICD codes has also been used to study resource utilization, such as for common procedures like adenotonsillectomies in different hospital settings and for rare entities like laryngotracheal separations.[56,57]

Pediatric health information system

Unlike KID, Pediatric Health Information System (PHIS) includes not only inpatient care but also services delivered in ambulatory surgery, observation, outpatient, and emergency settings from 45 free standing pediatric hospitals that are part of the Children's Hospital Association. Also different from KID, which is derived from administrative data, PHIS is considered a clinical registry database. The data from 1999 are longitudinal, meaning that patients can be tracked across multiple encounters. However, any care that occurs outside of the children's hospital system will not be captured by this database. While PHIS is representative of most tertiary or quaternary pediatric care, many hospitalized children receive care in nonchildren's hospital. It is unclear if PHIS accurately represents the care of common pediatric diagnoses in the community setting.

In otolaryngology, several studies have used PHIS to examine the utilization of care, readmission rates, and practice patterns for a wide range of uncommon diseases and procedures, including bilateral vocal fold immobility, esophageal atresia/tracheoesophageal fistula, and the Sistrunk procedure.[58-60] A recent study evaluated the accuracy of PHIS registry data in determining the surgical drainage rate of peritonsillar abscess compared to a retrospective chart review of the same cohort of patients.[61] They found that while there were some discrepancies, the accuracy of the PHIS database was relatively good. Misclassification that did occur was related to the underreporting of abscess drainage that was conducted outside of the operating room. In contrast to KID, which requires a fee for download of the data, access to PHIS is currently free of charge.

State databases

State ambulatory surgery services database/State emergency department database/State inpatient database

Another part of the HCUP program is a set of state-level databases that include the State Ambulatory Surgery Services Database (SASD), State Emergency Department Database (SEDD), and State Inpatient Database (SID).[62] SASD includes encounter-level data for ambulatory surgeries at hospital-owned facilities; SEDD captures emergency visits at hospital-owned emergency departments; and SID includes all inpatient care records in participating states. The SID captures an impressive number of hospital discharges, nearly 97% of all US community hospital discharges. This incorporates all nonfederal institutions including academic medical center, specialty hospitals, and pediatric hospitals. The SID provides the building blocks for the NIS, which is a nationwide database of hospital inpatient stays, as previously described.

There is a core file that contains core data elements including patient demographics, insurance, diagnoses, procedures, admission and discharge status, and length of stay. The SID can be linked to the American Hospital Association (AHA) Linkage File for more detailed hospital characteristics information for those states that allow the release of hospital identifiers. The HCUP Cost-to-Charge Ratio Files allow conversion of billed charges to hospital costs. The Diagnosis and Procedure Groups File is a discharge-level file that contains data elements designed to facilitate the use of the ICD diagnostic and procedure information in the core file. Data can be analyzed without sampling weights.

These state databases are well suited for research that requires complete enumeration of hospitals and discharges within a particular state. Researchers can use these databases to investigate questions unique to one state, compare data between states, and conduct research on a geographic region. In the otolaryngology literature, because these state databases capture most of the discharges in a given state, they have been used to examine practice patterns for various ambulatory surgeries.[63–66] However, they lack some detailed information about the surgery and complications. As with many administrative databases, the disease process cannot be further characterized beyond the diagnosis and procedure codes listed. It is important to note that certain data elements may not be available for every year, and that the available variables may vary across the different states. The results from state data also may not be generalizable to reflect overall national trends. These state databases are available after submission of an application and can be directly purchased through the HCUP website.[67]

Otolaryngology-specific databases
Creating healthcare excellence through education and research
Creating Healthcare Excellence through Education and Research (CHEER) created a database that stems solely from the otolaryngology practice-based network including community-based practices. The network comprises 30 provider sites in 19 states totaling more than 200 otolaryngologists.[68] The database captures 650,000 unique encounters from 260,000 unique patients from 2011 to 2013. Data are available at both the visit level and the patient level. The data are not intended to be nationally representative. It can be analyzed directly without applying sample weights.

Several studies have used the CHEER database to examine practice patterns among otolaryngologists for various diagnoses and procedures.[68–71] The utility of having an otolaryngology-specific database has also been studied previously. Although in NAMCS/NHAMCS, only 1.7% of visits were with otolaryngologists from 2005 to 2010. A comparative feasibility study conducted parallel analyses from the NAMCS/NHAMCS dataset and the CHEER dataset regarding the risk factors for pediatric sudden sensorineural hearing loss within a 1-year time span.[72] There were 14 SNHL patients identified from the NAMCS/NHAMCS, compared to 4623 from the CHEER database. Similarly, the number of observations for each of the common otolaryngology diagnoses, including chronic otitis media, Meniere's disease, cholesteatoma, adenoid hypertrophy, and turbinate hypertrophy, for 1 year in CHEER far surpassed those in NAMCS/NHAMCS, which were all under 30. The authors concluded that for specific inquiries pertaining to otolaryngology, databases that are not specific to otolaryngology may not have enough observations for sufficient analysis. This is especially true for NAMCS/NHAMCS as it employs a weighted system; if the number of observations does not meet the minimal criteria (aka 30), reliable conclusions cannot be drawn from the data.

There are a few disadvantages to using CHEER. The use of the database is limited to being part of the network, so it is not publicly available. The database only contains demographics, diagnoses, and procedures-related variables. It is also subject to inherent referral bias, as the CHEER draws data only from otolaryngologist-specific practices.[73] It is possible that there is a higher prevalence or severity of a disease among patients who are referred to specialists.[73] Further applications of the data from the CHEER network remain to be seen, and it is likely to be supplanted by the Reg-ent clinical data registry.

Reg-ent clinical data registry

Reg-ent is a clinical registry that was developed by the American Academy of Otolaryngology Head and Neck Surgery Foundation (AAO-HNS) in 2016. The goal of Reg-ent is to improve the quality of care and patient outcomes by compiling quality measures from otolaryngologists in various practice types and locations.[74] The registry pools data from private practice and academic settings across different geographic regions of the county. The registry has now grown to include over 2000 clinicians and is expected to continue to grow more dramatically. The information in the registry can be used to compare individual performances with national benchmarks and can help guide the AAO-HNS form improved guidelines for patient care. Efforts are underway to promote the use of the datasets for research opportunities.

Conclusion

Large databases provide researchers access to a large patient population with more nationally representative data than single institutional studies. In this sense, it serves as a powerful tool for epidemiologic and quality of care research. Despite its clear merits, there are limitations that must be considered, including the potential for data inaccuracy and bias. Each database has its unique advantages and drawbacks that need to be carefully considered before choosing the right database to address specific research questions. Critical appraisal of administrative database studies is important to avoid arriving at inaccurate conclusions.

References

1. Subbarayan RS, Koester L, Villwock MR, Villwock J. Proliferation and contributions of national database studies in otolaryngology literature published in the United States: 2005–2016. *Ann Otol Rhinol Laryngol.* September 2018;127(9):643–648. https://doi.org/10.1177/0003489418784968.

2. Bilimoria KY, Stewart AK, Winchester DP, Ko CY. The National Cancer Data Base: a powerful initiative to improve cancer care in the United States. *Ann Surg Oncol.* March 2008;15(3):683–690. https://doi.org/10.1245/s10434-007-9747-3.

3. Lenzi R, Fortunato S, Muscatello L. Top-cited articles of the last 30 years (1985–2014) in otolaryngology—head and neck surgery. *J Laryngol Otol.* February 2016;130(2):121–127. https://doi.org/10.1017/S002221511500300X.

4. Hoffman HT, Porter K, Karnell LH, et al. Laryngeal cancer in the United States: changes in demographics, patterns of care, and survival. *Laryngoscope.* September 2006;116(9 Pt 2 Suppl 111):1–13. https://doi.org/10.1097/01.mlg.0000236095.97947.26.

5. Alluri RK, Leland H, Heckmann N. Surgical research using national databases. *Ann Transl Med.* October 2016;4(20):393. https://doi.org/10.21037/atm.2016.10.49.

6. Haut ER, Pronovost PJ, Schneider EB. Limitations of administrative databases. *JAMA.* June 27, 2012;307(24):2589–2590. https://doi.org/10.1001/jama.2012.6626.

7. Stulberg JJ, Haut ER. Practical guide to surgical data sets: healthcare cost and utilization project national inpatient sample (NIS). *JAMA Surg.* 2018;153(6):586–587. https://doi.org/10.1001/jamasurg.2018.0542.

8. Golinvaux NS, Bohl DD, Basques BA, Grauer JN. Administrative database concerns: accuracy of International Classification of Diseases, Ninth Revision coding is poor for preoperative anemia in patients undergoing spinal fusion. *Spine.* November 15, 2014;39(24):2019–2023. https://doi.org/10.1097/BRS.0000000000000598.

9. Boudreaux M, Gangopadhyaya A, Long SK, Karaca Z. Using data from the healthcare cost and utilization project for state health policy research. *Med Care.* 2019;57(11):855–860. https://doi.org/10.1097/MLR.0000000000001196.

10. Bekkers S, Bot AG, Makarawung D, Neuhaus V, Ring D. The national hospital discharge survey and nationwide inpatient sample: the databases used affect results in THA research. *Clin Orthop Relat Res.* November 2014;472(11):3441–3449. https://doi.org/10.1007/s11999-014-3836-y.

11. Bur AM, Villwock MR, Nallani R, et al. National database research in head and neck reconstructive surgery: a call for increased transparency and reproducibility. *Otolaryngol Head Neck Surg.* 2021;164(2):315–321. https://doi.org/10.1177/0194599820938044.

12. Khera R, Krumholz HM. With great power comes great responsibility: big data research from the national inpatient sample. *Circ Cardiovasc Qual Outcomes.* 2017;10(7). https://doi.org/10.1161/CIRCOUTCOMES.117.003846.

13. Producing National HCUP Estimates - Accessible Version. *Healthcare Cost and Utilization Project (HCUP).* Rockville, MD: Agency for Healthcare Research and Quality;

December 2018. www.hcup-us.ahrq.gov/tech_assist/nationalestimates/508_course/508course_2018.jsp.

14. Ren Y, Sethi RKV, Stankovic KM. National trends in surgical resection of vestibular schwannomas. *Otolaryngol Head Neck Surg*. 2020;163(6):1244−1249. https://doi.org/10.1177/0194599820932148.

15. Khera R, Angraal S, Couch T, et al. Adherence to methodological standards in research using the national inpatient sample. *JAMA*. 2017;318(20):2011−2018. https://doi.org/10.1001/jama.2017.17653.

16. Khuri SF, Daley J, Henderson W, et al. The Department of Veterans Affairs' NSQIP: the first national, validated, outcome-based, risk-adjusted, and peer-controlled program for the measurement and enhancement of the quality of surgical care. National VA Surgical Quality Improvement Program. *Ann Surg*. October 1998;228(4):491−507. https://doi.org/10.1097/00000658-199810000-00006.

17. Velanovich V, Rubinfeld I, Patton JH, Ritz J, Jordan J, Dulchavsky S. Implementation of the national surgical quality improvement program: critical steps to success for surgeons and hospitals. *Am J Med Qual*. 2009;24(6):474−479. https://doi.org/10.1177/1062860609339937.

18. Stachler RJ, Yaremchuk K, Ritz J. Preliminary NSQIP results: a tool for quality improvement. *Otolaryngol Head Neck Surg*. July 2010;143(1):26−30. https://doi.org/10.1016/j.otohns.2010.02.017.

19. Raval MV, Pawlik TM. Practical guide to surgical data sets: national surgical quality improvement program (NSQIP) and pediatric NSQIP. *JAMA Surg*. 2018;153(8):764−765. https://doi.org/10.1001/jamasurg.2018.0486.

20. Lucas DJ, Haut ER, Hechenbleikner EM, Wick EC, Pawlik TM. Avoiding immortal time bias in the American College of surgeons national surgical quality improvement program readmission measure. *JAMA Surg*. August 2014;149(8):875−877. https://doi.org/10.1001/jamasurg.2014.115.

21. Patel VA, Khaku A, Carr MM. Pediatric thyroidectomy: NSQIP-P analysis of adverse perioperative outcomes. *Ann Otol Rhinol Laryngol*. April 2020;129(4):326−332. https://doi.org/10.1177/0003489419889069.

22. Kordahi AM, Hoppe IC, Lee ES. A comparison of free tissue transfers to the head and neck performed by sugeons and otolaryngologists. *J Craniofac Surg*. 2016;27(1):e82−e85. https://doi.org/10.1097/SCS.0000000000002240.

23. Schneider AL, Deig CR, Prasad KG, et al. Ability of the national surgical quality improvement program risk calculator to predict complications following total laryngectomy. *JAMA Otolaryngol Head Neck Surg*. 2016;142(10):972−979. https://doi.org/10.1001/jamaoto.2016.1809.

24. Lawson EH, Louie R, Zingmond DS, et al. A comparison of clinical registry versus administrative claims data for reporting of 30-day surgical complications. *Ann Surg*. December 2012;256(6):973−981. https://doi.org/10.1097/SLA.0b013e31826b4c4f.

25. Prasad KG, Nelson BG, Deig CR, Schneider AL, Moore MG. ACS NSQIP risk calculator: an accurate predictor of complications in major head and neck surgery? *Otolaryngol Head Neck Surg*. 2016;155(5):740−742. https://doi.org/10.1177/0194599816655976.

26. Ma Y, Laitman BM, Patel V, et al. Assessment of the NSQIP surgical risk calculator in predicting microvascular head and neck reconstruction outcomes. *Otolaryngol Head Neck Surg*. 2019;160(1):100−106. https://doi.org/10.1177/0194599818789132.

27. Sheils CR, Dahlke AR, Kreutzer L, Bilimoria KY, Yang AD. Evaluation of hospitals participating in the American College of surgeons national surgical quality improvement program. *Surgery*. 2016;160(5):1182−1188. https://doi.org/10.1016/j.surg.2016.04.034.

28. Jones EA, Shuman AG, Egleston BL, Liu JC. Common pitfalls of head and neck research using cancer registries. *Otolaryngol Head Neck Surg.* 2019;161(2):245−250. https://doi.org/10.1177/0194599819838823.
29. Merkow RP, Rademaker AW, Bilimoria KY. Practical guide to surgical data sets: national cancer database (NCDB). *JAMA Surg.* 2018;153(9):850−851. https://doi.org/10.1001/jamasurg.2018.0492.
30. Boffa DJ, Rosen JE, Mallin K, et al. Using the national cancer database for outcomes research: a review. *JAMA Oncol.* 2017;3(12):1722−1728. https://doi.org/10.1001/jamaoncol.2016.6905.
31. Megwalu UC, Sirjani D, Devine EE. Oropharyngeal squamous cell carcinoma incidence and mortality trends in the United States, 1973−2013. *Laryngoscope.* 2018;128(7):1582−1588. https://doi.org/10.1002/lary.26972.
32. Turner JH, Richmon JD. Head and neck rhabdomyosarcoma: a critical analysis of population-based incidence and survival data. *Otolaryngol Head Neck Surg.* December 2011;145(6):967−973. https://doi.org/10.1177/0194599811417063.
33. Martin E, Radomski S, Harley E. Sarcomas of the paranasal sinuses: an analysis of the SEER database. *Laryngoscope Investig Otolaryngol.* February 2019;4(1):70−75. https://doi.org/10.1002/lio2.245.
34. Janz TA, Graboyes EM, Nguyen SA, et al. A comparison of the NCDB and SEER database for research involving head and neck cancer. *Otolaryngol Head Neck Surg.* 2019;160(2):284−294. https://doi.org/10.1177/0194599818792205.
35. Jairam V, Park HS. Strengths and limitations of large databases in lung cancer radiation oncology research. *Transl Lung Cancer Res.* September 2019;8(Suppl 2):S172−S183. https://doi.org/10.21037/tlcr.2019.05.06.
36. Noone AM, Lund JL, Mariotto A, et al. Comparison of SEER treatment data with Medicare claims. *Med Care.* September 2016;54(9):e55−e64. https://doi.org/10.1097/MLR.0000000000000073.
37. Kumar A, Guss ZD, Courtney PT, et al. Evaluation of the use of cancer registry data for comparative effectiveness research. *JAMA Netw Open.* 2020;3(7):e2011985. https://doi.org/10.1001/jamanetworkopen.2020.11985.
38. Curtin LR, Mohadjer LK, Dohrmann SM, et al. The national health and nutrition examination survey: sample design, 1999−2006. *Vital Health Stat 2.* May 2012;(155):1−39.
39. Zipf G, Chiappa M, Porter KS, Ostchega Y, Lewis BG, Dostal J. National health and nutrition examination survey: plan and operations, 1999−2010. *Vital Health Stat 1.* August 2013;(56):1−37.
40. Johnson CL, Dohrmann SM, Burt VL, Mohadjer LK. National health and nutrition examination survey: sample design, 2011−2014. *Vital Health Stat 2.* March 2014;(162):1−33.
41. Johnson CL, Paulose-Ram R, Ogden CL, et al. National health and nutrition examination survey: analytic guidelines, 1999−2010. *Vital Health Stat 2.* September 2013;(161):1−24.
42. McManus B, Harbarger C, Grillis A, et al. Otoscopy and tympanometry outcomes from the national health and nutrition examination survey (NHANES). *Am J Otolaryngol.* 2022;43(2):103332. https://doi.org/10.1016/j.amjoto.2021.103332.
43. Choi JS, Yu AJ, Voelker CCJ, Doherty JK, Oghalai JS, Fisher LM. Prevalence of tinnitus and associated factors among Asian Americans: results from a national sample. *Laryngoscope.* 2020;130(12):E933−E940. https://doi.org/10.1002/lary.28535.
44. Juszczak H, Aubin-Pouliot A, Sharon JD, Loftus PA. Sinonasal risk factors for eustachian tube dysfunction: cross-sectional findings from NHANES 2011−2012. *Int Forum Allergy Rhinol.* 2019;9(5):466−472. https://doi.org/10.1002/alr.22275.

45. Hoffman HJ, Dobie RA, Losonczy KG, Themann CL, Flamme GA. Declining prevalence of hearing loss in US adults aged 20 to 69 years. *JAMA Otolaryngol Head Neck Surg.* 2017;143(3):274−285. https://doi.org/10.1001/jamaoto.2016.3527.

46. Goshtasbi K, Abouzari M, Risbud A, et al. Tinnitus and subjective hearing loss are more common in migraine: a cross-sectional NHANES analysis. *Otol Neurotol.* 2021;42(9): 1329−1333. https://doi.org/10.1097/MAO.0000000000003247.

47. Hill SC, Zuvekas SH, Zodet MW. Implications of the accuracy of MEPS prescription drug data for health services research. *Inquiry.* 2011;48(3):242−259. https://doi.org/10.5034/inquiryjrnl_48.03.04.

48. Kravietz A, Angara P, Le M, Sargi Z. Disparities in screening for head and neck cancer: evidence from the NHANES, 2011−2014. *Otolaryngol Head Neck Surg.* April 2018; 159:683−691. https://doi.org/10.1177/0194599818773074.

49. Fleming-Dutra KE, Hersh AL, Shapiro DJ, et al. Prevalence of inappropriate antibiotic prescriptions among US ambulatory care visits, 2010−2011. *JAMA.* 2016;315(17): 1864−1873. https://doi.org/10.1001/jama.2016.4151.

50. Aparasu RR, Rege S. National surveys to evaluate prescribing practices: methodological considerations. *Res Social Adm Pharm.* 2022;18(2):2317−2324. https://doi.org/10.1016/j.sapharm.2021.06.020.

51. Smith SS, Kern RC, Chandra RK, Tan BK, Evans CT. Variations in antibiotic prescribing of acute rhinosinusitis in United States ambulatory settings. *Otolaryngol Head Neck Surg.* May 2013;148(5):852−859. https://doi.org/10.1177/0194599813479768.

52. Mattos JL, Woodard CR, Payne SC. Trends in common rhinologic illnesses: analysis of U.S. healthcare surveys 1995−2007. *Int Forum Allergy Rhinol.* 2011;1(1):3−12. https://doi.org/10.1002/alr.20003.

53. Corkum KS, Baumann LM, Lautz TB. Complication rates for pediatric hepatectomy and nephrectomy: a comparison of NSQIP-P, PHIS, and KID. *J Surg Res.* 2019;240: 182−190. https://doi.org/10.1016/j.jss.2019.03.005.

54. Favre N, Patel VA, Carr MM. Complications in pediatric acute mastoiditis: HCUP KID analysis. *Otolaryngol Head Neck Surg.* 2021;165(5):722−730. https://doi.org/10.1177/0194599821989633.

55. Amoils M, Chang KW, Saynina O, Wise PH, Honkanen A. Postoperative complications in pediatric tonsillectomy and adenoidectomy in ambulatory vs inpatient settings. *JAMA Otolaryngol Head Neck Surg.* April 2016;142(4):344−350. https://doi.org/10.1001/jamaoto.2015.3634.

56. McCormick ME, Fissenden TM, Chun RH, Lander L, Shah RK. Resource utilization and national demographics of laryngotracheal trauma in children. *JAMA Otolaryngol Head Neck Surg.* September 2014;140(9):829−832. https://doi.org/10.1001/jamaoto.2014.1410.

57. Raol N, Zogg CK, Boss EF, Weissman JS. Inpatient pediatric tonsillectomy: does hospital type affect cost and outcomes of care? *Otolaryngol Head Neck Surg.* March 2016; 154(3):486−493. https://doi.org/10.1177/0194599815621739.

58. Brooks JA, Cunningham MJ, Hughes AL, Kawai K, Dombrowski ND, Adil E. Postoperative disposition following pediatric Sistrunk procedures: a national database query. *Laryngoscope.* 2021;131(7):E2352−E2355. https://doi.org/10.1002/lary.29331.

59. Patterson K, Beyene TJ, Asti L, Althubaiti A, Lind M, Pattisapu P. Quantifying upper aerodigestive sequelae in esophageal atresia/tracheoesophageal fistula neonates. *Laryngoscope.* 2022;132(3):695−700. https://doi.org/10.1002/lary.29798.

60. Shay AD, Zaniletti I, Davis KP, Bolin E, Richter GT. Characterizing pediatric bilateral vocal fold dysfunction: analysis with the pediatric health information system database. *Laryngoscope*. July 07, 2022;133:1228–1233. https://doi.org/10.1002/lary.30274.

61. Chisholm AG, Little BD, Johnson RF. Validating peritonsillar abscess drainage rates using the Pediatric hospital information system data. *Laryngoscope*. 2020;130(1): 238–241. https://doi.org/10.1002/lary.27836.

62. HCUP Databases. *Healthcare Cost and Utilization Project (HCUP)*. Rockville, MD: Agency for Healthcare Research and Quality; September 2021. www.hcup-us.ahrq. gov/sasdoverview.jsp.

63. Orosco RK, Lin HW, Bhattacharyya N. Safety of adult ambulatory direct laryngoscopy: revisits and complications. *JAMA Otolaryngol Head Neck Surg*. August 2015;141(8): 685–689. https://doi.org/10.1001/jamaoto.2015.1172.

64. Ference EH, Graber M, Conley D, et al. Operative utilization of balloon versus traditional endoscopic sinus surgery. *Laryngoscope*. January 2015;125(1):49–56. https://doi.org/10.1002/lary.24901.

65. Soneru CP, Pinto JM. Patient and surgeon factors explain variation in the frequency of frontal sinus surgery. *Laryngoscope*. 2018;128(9):2008–2014. https://doi.org/10.1002/lary.27115.

66. Bhattacharyya N. Ambulatory sinus and nasal surgery in the United States: demographics and perioperative outcomes. *Laryngoscope*. March 2010;120(3):635–638. https://doi.org/10.1002/lary.20777.

67. HCUP Data Use Training. *Healthcare Cost and Utilization Project (HCUP)*. Rockville, MD: Agency for Healthcare Research and Quality; September 2022. www.hcup-us.ahrq. gov/tech_assist/dua.jsp.

68. Schulz KA, Esmati E, Godley FA, et al. Patterns of migraine disease in otolaryngology: a CHEER network study. *Otolaryngol Head Neck Surg*. 2018;159(1):42–50. https://doi.org/10.1177/0194599818764387.

69. Chapurin N, Pynnonen MA, Roberts R, et al. CHEER national study of chronic rhinosinusitis practice patterns: disease comorbidities and factors associated with surgery. *Otolaryngol Head Neck Surg*. 2017;156(4):751–756. https://doi.org/10.1177/0194599817691476.

70. Lee WT, Witsell DL, Parham K, et al. Tonsillectomy bleed rates across the CHEER practice research network: pursuing guideline adherence and quality improvement. *Otolaryngol Head Neck Surg*. 2016;155(1):28–32. https://doi.org/10.1177/0194599816630523.

71. Witsell DL, Mulder H, Rauch S, Schulz KA, Tucci DL. Steroid use for sudden sensorineural hearing loss: a CHEER network study. *Otolaryngol Head Neck Surg*. 2018; 159(5):895–899. https://doi.org/10.1177/0194599818785142.

72. Bellmunt AM, Roberts R, Lee WT, et al. Does an otolaryngology-specific database have added value? A comparative feasibility analysis. *Otolaryngol Head Neck Surg*. 2016; 155(1):56–64. https://doi.org/10.1177/0194599816651036.

73. Nelson LM, Franklin GM, Hamman RF, Boteler DL, Baum HM, Burks JS. Referral bias in multiple sclerosis research. *J Clin Epidemiol*. 1988;41(2):187–192. https://doi.org/10.1016/0895-4356(88)90093-5.

74. Denneny JC. Regent: a new otolaryngology clinical data registry. *Otolaryngol Head Neck Surg*. 2016;155(1):5. https://doi.org/10.1177/0194599816651585x.

Sources of high-dimensional data—The electronic health record, health systems, and insurance and payor data

Molly P. Jarman, PhD, MPH [1], Rohith (Reddy) Kariveda, BA [2], Robert S. Semco, BS [3], Jennifer J. Shin, MD, SM [4]

[1]*Center for Surgery and Public Health, Department of Surgery, Brigham and Women's Hospital, Boston, MA, United States;* [2]*Boston University Chobanian and Avedisian School of Medicine, Boston, MA, United States;* [3]*Harvard Medical School, Boston, MA USA;* [4]*Department of Otolaryngology - Head and Neck Surgery, Harvard Medical School, Boston, MA, United States*

Data-driven medical care supports optimal treatment plans. In order to provide the data which drives these decisions, we evaluate patient outcomes, ideally in large populations. When exploring clinical questions, researchers may access patient data from a variety of sources.

Researchers may choose to use **primary data** sources, which involves data collection for the sole purpose of that study. Primary data sources may present several advantages, including increased probability of completeness, validity, and reliability; they may also be advantageous in that researchers who collected and inputted the data are also performing the analysis.[1] Primary data sources, however, also have disadvantages. For example, the data collection process may be time-consuming, costly, and labor-intensive. Even if proper steps are taken, it may ultimately be difficult to scale to sample sizes which support adequate power.

Beyond primary data, there are often large preexisting pools of patient information that may be repurposed for clinical research. Referred to as **secondary data**, these sources often offer a size and accessibility advantage over primary data.[2] There are several common sources of secondary data used in surgical outcomes and health services research, including insurance and payment records, electronic health records (EHRs), surveys, registries, and datasets from other existing research studies. Each source offers a unique set of advantages, disadvantages, and applications to clinical research.

Within this chapter, key sources, elements, and strategies of secondary data research will be discussed in detail. We begin by introducing common sources for database research, focusing specifically on secondary data sources such as insurance and payment databases, EHRs, surveys, and health registries. National Ambulatory

Big Data in Otolaryngology. https://doi.org/10.1016/B978-0-443-10520-3.00003-4

Medical Care Survey (NAMCS)/National Hospital Ambulatory Medical Care Survey (NHAMCS) and Reg-ent, a national ambulatory survey and a medical specialty-specific registry respectively, are also discussed in detail to provide specific context for the uses, advantages, and disadvantages of common surgical data sources. Tables are included throughout the chapter with commonly used examples of each secondary database type to provide further insight on the applications of these sources. We also discuss logistical and data access aspects which support strong practices in handling of patient information. In addition, the chapter describes measures used to classify patients and cases in clinical studies which allow researchers to best discern relationships between cause-and-effect variables. Finally, we conclude with a summarized overview to provide key takeaways for this material.

Insurance and payment databases

Insurance and payment databases are among the most widely used secondary data sources for surgical outcomes and health services research. These resources typically include data on diagnoses, procedures, and patient demographics. In many cases, they can be linked with other sources, integrating data on hospital and physician characteristics, community sociodemographics, and even historic events. Insurance and payment datasets contained structured data, typically following standard coding taxonomies like the *International Statistical Classification of Diseases and Related Health Problems* (ICD) or *Current Procedural Terminology* (CPT). Table 3.1 describes insurance and payment databases commonly used in research.

One of the primary benefits of insurance and payment databases is their longitudinal nature. Many databases allow researchers to track individual patients' healthcare encounters over time, constructing a timeline of diagnosis, treatment, and outcomes. Prospective collection of longitudinal data is logistically cost prohibitive. Insurance and payment databases offer a cost-effective alternative. Insurance and payment databases are typically very large, representing millions of individual patients, making them useful when studying rare conditions or events. Additionally, many insurance and payment databases contain information from, or can be linked with, the American Hospital Association annual survey, incorporating data on hospital size, service lines, and financial status. Insurance databases containing patients' residential zip code can be linked with community-level sociodemographic characteristics or other measures of geographic access to care, and databases with National Provider Identifiers (NPIs) can be linked with data on clinician specialty, training, and work experience.

While insurance and payment data offer a wealth of data, operationalizing payment data into meaningful variables for research can be a challenge. Researchers planning to use insurance and payment are best served by thoughtfully outlining the variables needed to meet their research objectives, and by using validated methods to create variables of interest from available data. For example, researchers

Table 3.1 Commonly used insurance and payment databases.

Database name	Brief description	Key data elements included	Key data elements *not included*
Medicare Claims	National dataset of enrollment data, fee-for-service claims, and encounter-level data for Medicare beneficiaries.	Patient demographics Enrollment in Medicare Diagnoses Procedures Disposition Medications Durable medical equipment Home health services Hospice services Expenditures	Laboratory and imaging results Clinician notes
Commercial Insurance (Optum, Marketscan)	Longitudinal datasets of enrollment data, insurance claims, and more. Built from private insurance, but may also include some Medicare and Medicaid data.	Patient demographics Insurance type Diagnoses Procedures Disposition Medications Durable medical equipment Home health services Hospice services Expenditures Laboratory results (for a subset of patients)	Clinician notes
HCUP National Datasets	Nationally representative sample containing encounter-level data on inpatient discharges, ambulatory surgeries, and emergency department visits.	Varies by year and dataset Patient demographic Payer type Diagnoses Procedures Hospital identifiers Charges Geographic region	Deidentified patient identifiers Patient ZIP code American hospital association ID Expenditures Longitudinal information on individual patients Private insurance type Clinician notes

Continued

Table 3.1 Commonly used insurance and payment databases.—*cont'd*

Database name	Brief description	Key data elements included	Key data elements *not* included
HCUP State Datasets	State-specific datasets containing encounter-level data for all inpatient discharges, hospital-owned ambulatory surgeries and services, and emergency department visits.	Varies by year, state, and dataset Deidentified patient identifiers Patient demographics Payer type Diagnoses Procedures Hospital identifiers Charges Geographic region Patient ZIP code AHA ID	Expenditures Longitudinal information on individual patients Private insurance type Clinician notes
All Payer Claims Data	State-specific datasets containing medical, dental, and pharmacy claims reported by payers.	Varies Deidentified patient identifiers Patient demographics Payer and contract type Diagnoses Procedures Physician characteristics Health plan characteristics Expenditures	Claims for uninsured patients Denied claims Laboratory and imaging results Clinician notes

who need to measure or account for risk of adverse outcomes attributable to comorbidities can calculate the Elixhauser Comorbidity Index using ICD codes.[3] Common methods for classifying patients based on diagnostic and procedure data are outlined subsequently in this chapter. Researchers should also be mindful of biases created by the structure of the US healthcare payment system. Insurance plans often require entry of diagnosis codes when ordering and paying for laboratory or imaging needed to "rule out" the diagnosis in question. Failure to account for this practice in research can lead to overestimates of disease prevalence. For example, a patient may periodically have a diagnosis of diabetes mellitus in their payment records, paired with orders for blood work to rule out insulin resistance. Researchers should refer to the literature to identify best practices for determining the presence of relevant diagnosis. In the absence of literature concerning methods for measuring construct of interest in insurance and payment data, researchers may need to complete a validation study of their own. Insurance and payment databases may also systematically exclude uninsured patients, which can bias results. States are increasingly developing All Payer Claims Databases as an alternative source of insurance and payment data that does include uninsured patients.

Electronic health records

EHRs are digital versions of patient's healthcare charts. Depending on the patient care setting, EHRs may contain information on diagnoses, treatment decisions, laboratory tests, imaging, clinical notes, and patient histories. EHRs are designed to meet the needs of healthcare providers in real-world settings, and contain both structured data (i.e., responses selected from a fixed set of options) and unstructured data (e.g., typed clinician notes).

The primary benefit of using EHR data for research is access to clinical data that are not typically available in claims- and payment-based datasets. Such data elements include laboratory values, imaging results, patient care notes, and histories. Data reported as discrete values, like laboratory values, are typically available in a structured format, making them relatively easy to use. Other forms of data, such as the standard patient care notes, typically require more effort to get to format data for research. Researchers who want to use unstructured data to assess variables that are not otherwise reflected in structured fields can manually extract data from EHR charts for smaller studies, or using computer-based extraction programs. For example, researchers in South Korea are using a technique called natural language processing to automatically extract thyroid cancer staging data from electronic patient charts, and populate a standardized data framework for studying long-term outcomes.[4]

In addition to data extraction efforts, accessing EHR data can be a challenge. Large academic medical centers may have established protocols for reviewing and approving research using EHR data, and may even provide data cleaning and formatting.

A limitation of EHR data is that researchers typically only have access to healthcare facilities affiliated with their own institution. While the Health Insurance Portability and Accountability Act (HIPAA) does allow healthcare organizations to share deidentified data with researchers, healthcare organizations have little incentive to undertake the time-consuming process of extracting, formatting, and cleaning data for researchers at outside institutions. Researchers who want to use EHR data from other institutions can consider working as coinvestigators. Data use agreements (DUAs) and research ethics reviews require thoughtful navigation, but the richness of data available is worth the effort.

- **Insurance and payment databases**—demographic, diagnostic, and procedural data on millions of patients organized by coding taxonomies; may be linked to external datasets
  - Advantages: allow the study of rare pathologies and consideration of several covariates versus disadvantages: difficulty operationalizing variables and potential for healthcare system biases
- **Electronic health records (EHRs)**—digital presentations of patient medical information
  - Advantages: contains data not available through insurance databases versus disadvantages: difficulty using unstructured data, potentially laborious data extraction process, and lack of access to EHR data from other institutions
- **Surveys**—structured and unstructured data from written questionnaires or spoken interviews
  - Advantages: contains data not available in insurance databases or EHRs versus disadvantages: sampling method may impact validity and generalizability, and may have to be supplemented with insurance databases or EHR data
  - **NAMCS and NHAMCS**—national ambulatory surveys distributed to nonfederal physicians and hospitals, respectively, to record patient data and generate weighted geographical aggregates
- **Registry data**—conglomerations of patient data from insurance databases, EHRs, or surveys based on specific criteria of interest
  - Advantages: useful to study rare conditions and are research-oriented with operationalized variables versus disadvantages: must pay for access, may forfeit certain rights to research findings
  - **Reg-ent**—otolaryngology-specific database that contains quality and performance e-Measures for clinical research, quality improvement, provider performance tracking, payer value, and continued licensure purposes
- **Additional steps to safely and effectively handle secondary data** may include the completion of DUAs between institutions, human research ethics review for sensitive health data research, extensive data storage and security measures, and the consultation of data managers and biostatisticians
- Patient outcomes may vary based on **exposure/independent variables and covariates. Disease severity, comorbidity, procedural risk, and sociodemographic variables** should be considered before making conclusions on the relationship between cause and outcome

Surveys

Survey data are collected prospectively through written questionnaires or interviews. Surveys may be conducted for a specific study or may be designed for general use in a wide range of research projects. The data elements contained in survey databases vary substantially, depending on the topic and purpose of the survey. Survey participants are typically selected through a specific recruitment protocol, which may include random selection from a defined population, as well as weighted sampling strategies to support generalizability of the data to a population of interest. Most survey data are structured, with response options determined during questionnaire development, although some surveys will have unstructured data requiring extraction or qualitative review. Table 3.2 describes survey databases commonly used for surgical outcome and health services research.

Table 3.2 Commonly used survey databases.

Database name	Brief description	Key data elements included	Key data elements *not* included
AHA Annual Survey	Financial, structural, and operational data provided by over 6200 hospitals	Organizational structure Facility location Facility type Services provided Bed counts Patient utilization Staffing Total expenses	Patient-level clinical data Facility revenue
National Health Interview Survey	Annual survey representative of US civilian population, with core and rotating topical questions	Demographics Comorbidities Health insurance Healthcare access/use Health behaviors Function/disability Service utilization Major diagnoses	Diagnoses of conditions not covered by survey
Health and Retirement Study	Longitudinal survey of adults age ≥50 can link with Medicare claims	Demographics Income Work/employment status Assets Pension plans Health insurance Disability Physical health/function Cognitive function Healthcare expenditures	Non-Medicare claims
National Health and Nutrition Examination Study	Annual Survey representative of US civilian population, including interview and physical exam data	Demographics Common comorbidities Sleep behavior Physical activity Diet Immunization status Nutritional status Environmental exposures	Identifiers to link records over time Clinical treatment

The primary benefit of survey data is the ability to measure constructs that are not reflected in insurance or EHR data. This includes patient-reported outcomes (e.g., health-related quality of life) and individual sociodemographic characteristics (e.g., education, immigration status, income). Some surveys are conducted longitudinally, allowing researchers to follow individual participants over time. Surveys can also include data from people who did not have a formal healthcare encounter. On occasion, surveys are linked with data from other sources, including EHRs and insurance records. This linkage enhances the quality of data analysis, and can support efforts to validate measures derived from diagnosis and procedure codes.

Researchers interested in using survey data in secondary analyses benefit from taking the time to query, understand, and vet the survey methodology. Considerations include:

- What was the original intent of the survey? This will influence decisions about patient inclusion and exclusion, as well as the structure and content of the data.
- How was the survey designed to have internal and external validity?
- Is the survey population representative of the population to which you want to generalize?
- Are there inclusion or exclusion criteria that might introduce bias into your analysis, such as selection based on a specific diagnosis or exclusion based on demographic characteristics?

In general, surveys conducted for a specific study will have generalizability limited to the population of interest in the original study. Surveys conducted for general use have broader generalizability, but may suffer from biases due to large-scale data collection techniques, including use of random digit dialing for phone interviewers, or convenience sampling.

National Ambulatory Medical Care Survey and National Hospital Ambulatory Medical Care Survey: General ambulatory databases

NAMCS is an annual national survey by the National Center for Health Statistics that looks at patient visits to physician offices. Each participating nonfederally employed physician is randomly assigned a 1-week period where patient encounters and drug data are electronically collected.[5,6] Similarly, NHAMCS is another annual national survey by the National Center for Health Statistics that examines ambulatory visits to emergency departments. Participating nonfederal, nonmilitary, and non-VA hospitals are sampled during a random 4-week period to collect patient data, visit details, and facility data. A three-stage probability sampling design is used for both surveys, and weighted locational aggregates are used to determine population estimates.[5,7] The results may be analyzed per year, per setting type, and per database, or both databases may be combined to increase reliability of population estimates.[8,9]

Ambulatory databases such as NAMCS and NHAMCS have advantages and disadvantages. For some subspecialty diseases, the databases may not have enough otolaryngology-specific data to support statistically significant analyses based on epidemiological standards.[10] For instance, only 1.7% of NAMCS data arises from visits to otolaryngologists, and it may therefore lack enough data points in certain instances.[10] However, NAMCS and NHAMCS have been used in several population-level otolaryngology studies, and are especially useful in studying common otolaryngological symptoms and diagnoses like chronic rhinosinusitis,[9] otitis media,[11] allergic rhinitis,[12] obstructive sleep apnea,[13] and gastroesophageal reflux disease (GERD).[13]

Registry data

Health registries are collections of data following individual patients over time, with enrollment based on a specific disease, procedure, or other exposure of interest. Registries may exist solely for research purposes, or may be mandated by public health authorities to monitor disease incidence and outcomes.[14] The exact data elements included vary widely from one registry to another, but you can generally expect to find data on diagnoses, procedures, disease staging, patient history, demographics, and long-term outcomes. Registries pull data from a variety of sources, including EHRs, insurance claims, and surveys. Table 3.3 describes data registries commonly used for surgical outcome and health services research.

Table 3.3 Commonly used registry databases.

Database name	Brief description	Key data elements included	Key data elements *not* included
SEER Cancer	Population-based registry of cancer incidence and survival data from 22 geographic areas representing 48% of the US population. Can be linked to Medicare claims, the Medicare Health Outcomes Survey, and the Consumer Assessment of Healthcare Providers and Systems.	Patient demographics Primary tumor site Tumor characteristics Treatment details Survival Expenditures (with Medicare claims) Complications (with Medicare claims)	Clinician notes
National Cancer Database	Hospital-based registry of cancer cases representing 72% of all newly diagnosed cancers in the US.	Patient demographics Primary tumor site Tumor characteristics Treatment details 30- and 90-day mortality Vital status, death, or last contact	Clinician notes Expenditures Complications
National Trauma Databank	National registry of trauma cases reported by level I–V or undesignated trauma centers for pediatric and adult patients.	Patient demographics Facility characteristics Injury type Vitals Procedures Comorbidities Outcomes (prehospital time, length of stay, complications)	Clinician notes Expenditures Laboratory results
National Surgical Quality Improvement Program	National registry of clinical and demographic data sourced from electronic medical records of a large sample of surgical patients.	Patient demographics Comorbidities Procedure Anesthesia technique Preoperative lab work Outcomes (length of stay, 30-day complications, readmissions, death)	Clinician notes Expenditures

Registries can be powerful sources of data for research, with the ability to study a wide range of long-term outcomes associated with disease risk factors and treatment decisions. Due to the targeted selection criteria and high participation rates, disease-specific registries are useful for rare diagnoses, exposures, and outcomes. As with surveys, registries often incorporate patient-reported outcomes and other data elements that are not available through insurance and payment data. Registries may also include data extracted from EHRs, reducing some of the data collection burden for future data users. Finally, registries typically take care of data cleaning, standardization, and operationalization of variables before sharing databases with researchers. This means researchers do not need to commit as much time and money to data preparation, and can begin substantive analysis sooner.

Similar to survey data, researchers should thoughtfully review the structure and content of registry data before pursuing substantive analysis. Registries can be rich sources of data, but often rely of EHR, insurance, and other secondary data sources, and the limitations of those sources then translate to the registries as well. Due to the time and effort required to compile registries, data access may require payment of fees or collaboration with registry investigators. Registries may also retain the right to complete research initiated by their own investigators, prior to sharing with outside investigators.

Reg-ent: An otolaryngology-specific registry

One such database, sponsored by the American Academy of Otolaryngology-Head and Neck Surgery, is Reg-ent. Reg-ent is an otolaryngology-specific patient registry with EHR-based data from 7,825,177 million unique patients and over 30 million patient encounters. These data have arisen from 1515 clinicians and over 500 practices.[15] The database has achieved Qualified Clinical Data Registry (QCDR) status since 2016, and ensures compliance with the reporting requirements from the Medicare Access and Children's Health Insurance Program Reauthorization Act (MACRA).[15,16] Reg-ent is subdivided into several subregistries, which can be accessed for a variety of purposes.

Primary uses: Advancing research, improving patient outcomes, and quality improvement

The Reg-ent database contains patient information which supports clinical effectiveness and outcomes research. Rich with data from both private practices and academic institutions, it is well suited to study the natural history and progression of disease, and ultimately care outcomes, especially for rare pathologies.[17] As Reg-ent grows, it can allow for the creation and reporting of risk-adjusted quality and performance e-Measures based on data, instead of de novo from guidelines and testing through beta phases.[18] The data may also be applied to facilitating the identification of eligible study candidates, ensuring adequate geographical coverage, and planning clinical trials.[17] By tracking patient data over time, the effectiveness of drugs and other pharmaceutical devices can also be monitored.[16]

Reg-ent is also positioned for quality improvement research, as it contains longitudinal data on patient outcomes and provider performance. Reg-ent's risk-adjusted quality measures can be divided into specialty-specific measures created by clinicians and broadly applicable measures that apply to several subspecialties.[15] Through long-term analyses of these measures, quality improvement can be measured, reported, and implemented as concordant with data-driven Clinical Practice Guidelines (CPG).[19]

Ancillary uses: Performance measurement, continued certification, and payer value

The Reg-ent registry may also be used for other purposes. Reg-ent quality measures are subdivided into Merit-based Incentive Payment System (MIPS) reportable measures, patient-reported performance/outcome measures, and "Test" measures (i.e. measures that have not yet been cleared for MIPS reporting, but can be used to evaluate physician performance). Comparing MIPS reportable measures or "Test" measures across providers and institutions can allow clinicians to identify shortcomings and improve practices.[15] With the involvement of the American Board of Otolaryngology, determination of points of improvement for specific providers may also impact the Maintenance of Certification process and the requirements for Maintenance of Licensure.[16]

Performance measures, a type of quality measure,[20] are also available to evaluate physician performance and performance gaps. These performance measures include de novo measures from the Reg-ent executive and advisory committees, CPG measures from guidelines, and previous Physician Quality Reporting System (PQRS) based measures. Different types of quality and performance measures from Reg-ent, including process and risk adjusted outcome measures, may inform payer value in MIPS reporting and Alternative Payer Models (APMs).[17]

Logistics and data access

Many investigators are surprised by the time and effort required to complete high-quality secondary data analyses. While secondary data analysis does eliminate the need for direct interaction with research participants, researchers still need to ensure data are handled securely, and that analyses are scientifically robust. Investigators may need to commit substantial effort to data extraction and preparation, or pay hefty fees to access data prepared by a third party. Before pursuing substantial secondary data projects, several key factors are worthy of consideration:

1) *Data use agreements*, or DUAs, are agreements between parties sharing data for research purposes. Typically, DUAs are signed by universities or research institutions on behalf of the investigators sharing and receiving data. This arrangement protects individual investigators from personal liability in the event data are mishandled, and also provides an extra level of oversight to ensure proposed data uses are legal and ethical. Widely used datasets, like Medicare claims or National Cancer Data Bank, have standard DUAs they will share with investigators requesting access to research data. Research institutions typically have a DUA template that they can adapt for data providers without an existing agreement draft. An institution's legal representative is typically responsible for reviewing and signing agreements.

2) *Human research ethics review* may or may not be required for a secondary data project, depending on the scope of data included. Research using healthcare data that are completely deidentified are usually exempt from review or not considered human subjects research. Nevertheless, secondary data research can have unforeseen ethical implications, and rules for secondary data use vary based on the original data source. It is good habit to submit all proposed secondary research protocols for institutional review board assessment for exemption or approval.

3) *Data storage and security* are often unexpected costs for secondary data research. Many datasets require secure storage above and beyond a password protected hard drive. DUAs for the most sensitive datasets may require a detailed data management plan outlining where data will be stored, who will have access and under what circumstances, how data access/use are monitored, and plans for data disposal at the end of the project. Deidentified data with minimal security requirements may still have substantial storage and processing requirements, far beyond what one would find in a desktop computer. Most large research institutions have information security and computing resources that can support projects using large databases.

4) *Biostatistician and data management experts* are valuable members of any research team completing secondary data analysis. Data managers are responsible for the acquisition, formatting, storage, and organization of large datasets. Depending on their training and research team needs, a data manager may also support data cleaning and extraction steps required to create discrete, project-specific analytic files. Biostatisticians generally have graduate-level training in statistics and/or epidemiology, and can execute analytic plans designed to test hypotheses. They can also provide guidance for study design, selection of statistical tests, and interpretation of results.

Coding taxonomy: Coding taxonomies are standardized approaches to classifying diagnoses, procedures, providers, and other commons elements reported in administrative data. Each code is associated with a unique data element, such as a diagnosis or procedure. Researchers who understand coding taxonomies can use these data to sort secondary data records into scientifically meaningful categories. Commonly used coding taxonomies include the International Classification of Disease, CPT, and CMS Provider Taxonomy Codes.

HIPAA, IRBs, and DUAs:
- The HIPAA outlines requirements for sharing healthcare data in the US. HIPAA allows secondary data research if the research has potential to benefit society at large, identifiers are removed before the research begins, and data handling procedure protects against unauthorized data access.
- Institutional review boards (IRBs) at research institutions ensure secondary data research projects are consistent with research ethics standards, including efforts to minimize risk of harm to research participants.
- DUAs are contracts between institutions providing and using secondary data for research. DUAs typically outline approved research use and data handling requirements.

General methods for classifying patients and cases

Selection of exposure variables and covariates is an important step when designed a secondary data project. Exposure, or independent, variables are the treatments or risk factors that are hypothesized to impact the outcome of interest. Covariates are characteristics of the patient, treatment, or environment that might impact the observed relationship between the exposure and outcome variable. As we mentioned in the section about insurance and payment data above, there are validated methods for measuring many exposures and covariates of interest for secondary data research.

Disease severity is a useful measure, both as an exposure for studies examining disease progression and outcomes and as a covariate in studies where disease severity might mask or change the relationship between exposure and outcome. Disease severity measures can vary based on the specific disease of interest, but generally categorize severity or stage of disease into four groups: (1) localized disease with low risk of complications, (2) regional disease and/or increase risk of complications, (3) disease impacting multiple sites/systems and with generally poor prognosis, and (4) disease likely to result in death.

Comorbidity indices are composite measures used to account for risk of poor outcomes attributed to diseases other than the one of interest in a study. For example, when examining the relationship between a patient referral policy and cancer outcomes, it is prudent to account for conditions which influence a patient outcome, such as diabetes or heart disease. The two most common indices are the Elixhauser Comorbidity Index[3] and the Charlson Comorbidity Index.[21] Both indices score patients based on the presence of selected comorbidities, with composite scores validated based on their ability to predicted mortality within 1 year. The Elixhauser index includes a wider range of comorbid conditions and generally performs better than Charlson.[22]

Procedural risk measures allow researchers to account for differences in the invasiveness, intensity, and overall risk or a surgical procedure when comparing outcomes in a heterogenous surgical population. At the highest level, procedures can be classified as major or minor, using Clinical Classifications Software (CCS)[23] from the Agency for Healthcare Research and Quality. CCS further classifies procedures based on anatomic location and disease treated. Statistical adjustment for CCS categories can help account for variability in outcomes attributable to the procedure itself, rather than the exposure of interest. Other procedure risk measures, such as the American Society of Anesthesiologists (ASA)[24] Classification System and the Acute Physiology and Chronic Health Evaluation (APACHE),[25] use patient health status characteristics to estimate the likelihood of adverse outcomes from a procedure. Unfortunately, many secondary data sources lack the data elements needed to calculate these scores.

Sociodemographic variables can meaningfully classify patients to improve our understanding of healthcare equity and disparities in outcomes. Most datasets include patient-level measures of age, sex, race, ethnicity, and health insurance status. Some may include measures of education, income, and preferred language. When patients' residential zip code or county are available, researchers can link patient-level data with community-level sociodemographic measures from the United State Census Bureau. These measures include basic population counts from the decennial census, as well as detailed data on the social and economic characteristics of populations from the American Community Survey.[26] Additionally, several validated measures of community-level risk exist, including the Social Vulnerability Index[27] and the Area Deprivation Index.[28] These composite measures account for the combined, competing, and collinear risks associated with multiple social determinants of health.

Survey sampling: Survey sampling protocols aim to maximize the generalizability of study results to the population of interest, while also minimizing bias caused by the sampling approach. Surveys intended for broad generalizability to the population at large frequently use stratified or weighted sampling approaches, ensuring the selected sample includes representation from key subpopulations. Probability sampling approaches randomly select participants from a defined sampling frame, such as using a random digit dialer to select a sample of phone numbers.

Summary overview

Insurance and payment databases: Insurance and payment databases contain patient demographic, diagnostic, and procedural data structured based on coding taxonomies. These databases contain longitudinal data from high volumes of patients, and may be linked with sources of information such as hospital or provider characteristics, along with socioeconomic variables. While there is often a plethora of data available in insurance and payment databases, operationalizing variables such as risk of adverse outcomes often requires substantial time and planning, as well as cognizance of potential biases introduced by the US healthcare system—overestimating disease prevalence using diagnostic codes and understudying uninsured patients are two common dangers encountered when using insurance and payment databases.

Electronic health records (EHRs): EHRs contain lab values, imaging, healthcare provider notes, referrals, and medical, familial, and social histories, which are typically not available in claims- or payment-based databases. While some structured data (e.g., lab values) may be easy to utilize for research purposes, other unstructured data (e.g., provider notes) can be cumbersome to work with. Unstructured data may be manually extracted for smaller studies, but larger studies may require the help of staff from academic centers or computerized extraction programs. Researchers often have access to EHR data only from their own institution, while requiring data use agreements between institutions for collaborative studies.

Surveys: Surveys contain both structured and unstructured prospective data from written or spoken questionnaires/interviews. Participants are generally chosen through random, convenience, weighted, or other sampling methods, which may impact study generalizability. Threats to internal and external validity may potentially occur if there are inclusion/exclusion criteria that cause the survey sample to be unrepresentative of your population of interest. Surveys can still be advantageous as they may contain data not typically available through insurance databases or EHRs, such as longitudinal changes in patient-reported outcome measures. Survey data may be linked with EHR or insurance record data to better support research claims.

National Ambulatory Medical Care Survey (NAMCS) and National Hospital Ambulatory Medical Care Survey (NHAMCS): These frequently used surveys include nonfederal physicians and hospitals from across the nation, and three-staged probability sampling is used to collect patient data, visit details, pharmaceutical data, and facility details into weighted locational aggregates. These databases can be used for population-level studies, especially for common conditions. However, their lack of exposure-specific data selection criteria may make them less applicable for fewer common conditions.

Registry data: Health registries enroll patients based on a specific criterion of interest, such as procedures, exposures, disease pathologies, or outcomes. They then track variables of interest over time. Registries may compile data from insurance databases, EHRs, and surveys, and therefore carry the same limitations as their aforementioned primary sources. They may exist for research, public health monitoring, quality assurance, and/or reimbursement purposes. Since they have a targeted selection criterion, they are useful to study risk factors and the efficacy of treatment decisions, even with rare diagnoses. Registries often contain research-grade, operationalized variables, making them handy for clinical studies. However, they may also require payment for access, and retain rights to complete any research done by their own participants.

Reg-ent: Reg-ent is an otolaryngology-specific database with EHR data from millions of patients and tens of millions of healthcare encounters. Tracking patient outcomes over time through quality and performance e-measures, Reg-ent provides a helpful tool for clinical and pharmaceutical research, especially in regards to rare head and neck diseases. It is also geared toward quality improvement and improving patient outcomes by allowing providers to track their own progress and compare it to the care decisions and outcomes of patients under other providers. Through MIPS-reportable measures, patient-reported performance measures, and continually developing "test" measures, Reg-ent is poised to measure provider performance as related to continued medical license certification and payer value/compensation.

Logistics and data access: Secondary data analyses often require additional steps to ensure that they are scientifically sound. Investigators may have to complete DUAs to share data between academic institutions or universities and protect themselves from personal liability in case of data mishandling. Human research ethics review may be required if the health data being studied is identifiable or sensitive. Even after review, researchers should be aware that there may be data storage and security measures that must be taken beyond a password-protected document or computer. Data managers and biostatisticians may be invaluable resources to support data extraction, cleaning, analysis, and interpretation.

General methods for classifying patients and cases: Exposure variables (i.e., independent variables) are conditions that change between patients, while covariates modify the effect between exposure and outcome variables. Disease severity, a measure which reflects the stage and seriousness of disease, may be used as an exposure or covariate variable. Comorbidity index scores account for covariate variables by considering conditions or factors outside of the diseases of interest that may impact a patient's ultimate health outcome. Procedural risk also accounts for effect modification by factoring in the risk of complications from a surgical procedure when analyzing surgical outcomes. It is also imperative that researchers consider sociodemographic variables, as they may have confounding effects on the relationship between exposure and outcome variables.

References

1. Gliklich RE, Dreyer NA, Leavy MB, eds. *Registries for Evaluating Patient Outcomes: A User's Guide*. 3rd ed. Agency for Healthcare Research and Quality (US); 2014. http://www.ncbi.nlm.nih.gov/books/NBK208616/. Accessed August 30, 2023.
2. Schlomer BJ, Copp HL. Secondary data analysis of large data sets in urology: successes and errors to avoid. *J Urol*. 2014;191(3):587−596. https://doi.org/10.1016/j.juro.2013.09.091.

3. Elixhauser A, Steiner C, Harris DR, Coffey RM. Comorbidity measures for use with administrative data. *Med Care*. 1998;36(1):8—27.

4. Yoo S, Yoon E, Boo D, et al. Transforming thyroid cancer diagnosis and staging information from unstructured reports to the observational medical outcome partnership common data model. *Appl Clin Inform*. 2022;13(3):521—531. https://doi.org/10.1055/s-0042-1748144.

5. NAMCS/NHAMCS - About the Ambulatory Health Care Surveys, Published December 30, 2021. https://www.cdc.gov/nchs/ahcd/about_ahcd.htm. Accessed 30 August 2023.

6. Ward BW, Myrick KL, Cherry DK. Physician specialty and office visits made by adults with diagnosed multiple chronic conditions: United States, 2014-2015. *Public Health Rep*. 2020;135(3):372—382. https://doi.org/10.1177/0033354920913005.

7. NHAMCS 2018-2020 Supporting Stat B 051118 - OMB 0920-0278. https://omb.report/icr/201809-0920-005/doc/86172601. Accessed 30 August 2023.

8. Hsiao J. *Understanding and Using NAMCS and NHAMCS Data*; 2010. https://www.cdc.gov/nchs/ppt/nchs2010/03_hsiao.pdf. Accessed June 29, 2022.

9. Gilani S, Pynnonen MA, Shin JJ. National practice patterns of antireflux Medication for chronic rhinosinusitis. *JAMA Otolaryngol Head Neck Surg*. 2016;142(7):627—633. https://doi.org/10.1001/jamaoto.2016.0937.

10. Bellmunt AM, Roberts R, Lee WT, et al. Does an otolaryngology-specific database have added value? A comparative feasibility analysis. *Otolaryngol Head Neck Surg*. 2016; 155(1):56—64. https://doi.org/10.1177/0194599816651036.

11. Prince AA, Rosenfeld RM, Shin JJ. Antihistamine use for otitis media with effusion: ongoing opportunities for quality improvement. *Otolaryngol Head Neck Surg*. 2015; 153(6):935—942. https://doi.org/10.1177/0194599815606709.

12. Roditi RE, Veling M, Shin JJ. Age: an effect modifier of the association between allergic rhinitis and Otitis media with effusion. *Laryngoscope*. 2016;126(7):1687—1692. https://doi.org/10.1002/lary.25682.

13. Gilani S, Quan SF, Pynnonen MA, Shin JJ. Obstructive sleep apnea and gastroesophageal reflux: a multivariate population-level analysis. *Otolaryngol Head Neck Surg*. 2016; 154(2):390—395. https://doi.org/10.1177/0194599815621557.

14. About NPCR | Cancer | CDC, Published August 16, 2023. https://www.cdc.gov/cancer/npcr/about.htm. Accessed 30 August 2023.

15. Meyer, J, Phatak, S, Caniano, E, Reg-ent Registry 101, (Presented at:).

16. Denneny JC. Regent: a new otolaryngology clinical data registry. *Otolaryngol Head Neck Surg*. 2016;155(1):5. https://doi.org/10.1177/0194599816651585.

17. Regent Leadership Team. Regent overview. In: *Presented at: American Academy of Otolaryngology - Head and Neck Surgery Annual Meeting*. 2021 (Alexandria, VA).

18. *Reg-EntSM Measures Presentation by Richard M. Rosenfeld, MD, MPH*; 2016. https://www.youtube.com/watch?v=tV6pHVNCgCU. Accessed August 30, 2023.

19. About Reg-ent, American Academy of Otolaryngology-Head and Neck Surgery (AAO-HNS). https://www.entnet.org/quality-practice/reg-ent-clinical-data-registry/about-reg-ent/. Accessed 30 August 2023.

20. Vila PM, Schneider JS, Piccirillo JF, Lieu JEC. Understanding quality measures in otolaryngology-head and neck surgery. *JAMA Otolaryngol Head Neck Surg*. 2016; 142(1):86—90. https://doi.org/10.1001/jamaoto.2015.2687.

21. Charlson ME, Pompei P, Ales KL, MacKenzie CR. A new method of classifying prognostic comorbidity in longitudinal studies: development and validation. *J Chronic Dis*. 1987;40(5):373—383. https://doi.org/10.1016/0021-9681(87)90171-8.

22. Sharabiani MTA, Aylin P, Bottle A. Systematic review of comorbidity indices for administrative data. *Med Care*. 2012;50(12):1109−1118. https://doi.org/10.1097/MLR.0b013e31825f64d0.

23. HCUP-US Tools and Software Page CCS-Services and Procedures. https://hcup-us.ahrq.gov/toolssoftware/ccs_svcsproc/ccssvcproc.jsp. Accessed 30 August 2023.

24. Doyle DJ, Hendrix JM, Garmon EH. American Society of Anesthesiologists Classification. In: *StatPearls*. StatPearls Publishing; 2023. http://www.ncbi.nlm.nih.gov/books/NBK441940/. Accessed August 30, 2023.

25. Acute Physiology and Chronic Health Evaluation (Apache) II Score − The Clinical Predictor in Neurosurgical Intensive Care Unit - PMC. https://www.ncbi.nlm.nih.gov/pmc/articles/PMC6629196/. Accessed 30 August 2023.

26. Bureau, UC, American Community Survey (ACS), Census.gov. https://www.census.gov/programs-surveys/acs. Accessed 30 August 2023.

27. CDC/ATSDR Social Vulnerability Index (SVI), Published July 12, 2023. https://www.atsdr.cdc.gov/placeandhealth/svi/index.html. Accessed 30 August 2023.

28. Maroko AR. Integrating social determinants of health with treatment and prevention: a new tool to assess local area deprivation. *Prev Chronic Dis*. 2016;13. https://doi.org/10.5888/pcd13.160221.

Best practices when interpreting big data studies: Considerations and red flags

Kelsey A. Duckett, MD[1] **and Evan M. Graboyes, MD, MPH**[1,2]

[1]*Department of Otolaryngology-Head and Neck Surgery, Medical University of South Carolina, Charleston, SC, United States;* [2]*Public Health Sciences, Medical University of South Carolina, Charleston, SC, United States*

Introduction

Between 2005 and 2016, there was a 10-fold increase in the number of "Big Data" studies published within the major otolaryngology journals.[1] These big data studies, which are based on clinical data housed in administrative databases, registries, or generated from the electronic health record (EHR), are also increasing in frequency in the biomedical literature writ large. From 2013 to 2020, the amount of data generated about health care delivery each year grew more than 15-fold.[2] From 1950 to 2020, the doubling time of medical knowledge decreased from 50 years to just 73 days; otolaryngologists completing residency in 2020 experienced four doublings in knowledge during their years of medical school and training. Clinicians are expected to provide high-quality care for patients using evidence-based practices. To do this effectively, clinicians must stay up-to-date on and understand the best-available research in their field and integrate this new knowledge with their own experience and patient's wishes when making clinical decisions.[3] Thoughtful interpretation of high-quality research is thus important to translating study findings into evidence-based clinical practices. Within the context of an unprecedented surge in published research, especially in emerging fields such as big data and associated highly sophisticated analyses, the continual task of interpreting and applying findings can feel overwhelming.[4,5]

Studies based on big data in otolaryngology have potential to inform clinical practice and improve patient outcomes. Many studies in otolaryngology have leveraged large datasets from clinical and/or administrative sources representing millions of patients. As more people engage in technologies and services that track their individual biometric data, studies investigating these data will become increasingly common. Such studies are useful for (1) representing routine clinical practice and analyzing real-world effectiveness of practices; (2) studying healthcare patterns, resources, cost, utilization, and disparities; and (3) exploring rare disease processes or

Big Data in Otolaryngology. https://doi.org/10.1016/B978-0-443-10520-3.00006-X

outcomes.[6] Additional big data opportunities include using genomic, proteomic, and metabolic data to (1) predict treatment response, (2) identify candidate disease markers, and (3) discover therapeutic targets. Although randomized clinical trials are vital to investigating the safety and efficacy of different treatments, they rarely offer evidence of practical utility and feasibility in the "real world." Big data studies help address this gap, allowing for the evaluation of safety and clinical effectiveness of therapies in routine clinical practice.[7]

Despite their importance, studies utilizing big data have important limitations that clinicians should be aware of. **These limitations, although present to some degree in all types of clinical research, are particularly salient within the context of big data**. This important caveat was reinforced recently when two big data studies, published only months apart in the same journal, investigated the same clinical question using data from the same database, yet arrived at different conclusions.[2,8,9] Both studies asked the same question: Do surgical retrieval bags decrease surgical site infections in patients undergoing laparoscopic appendectomy? Both studies also utilized data from the American College of Surgeons (ACS) National Surgical Quality Improvement Program (NSQIP) from the same year. However, the studies differed slightly in their eligibility criteria in forming study cohorts, definition of the outcome of interest, covariates, and analytic approaches. As a result, one study concluded that retrieval bags were associated with decreased surgical site infections in laparoscopic appendectomy (OR $= 0.6$, 95% CI 0.42 to 0.95, $P = .03$), while the other study concluded that retrieval bags were not associated with surgical site infections (OR $= 1.15$, 95% CI 0.78 to 1.69, $P = .49$).[2,8,9] As if the conflicting results were not perplexing enough to guide clinical practice, an accompanying viewpoint from Childers et al. argued that any study using the NSQIP database to address this clinical question would be severely limited because retrieval bag use is not reliably captured in the NSQIP dataset.[2,10] This example shows the potential pitfalls of applying big data to clinical practice if readers are not aware of the limitations of each database or able to critically evaluate methods utilized by researchers. It also highlights how big data research can be applicable to clinical practice and why it is important for clinicians to be aware of limitations when interpreting these studies.

To help the practicing otolaryngologist understand the promise of big data studies to inform clinical practice and understand their potential limitations, this chapter will describe considerations and potential red flags to guide best practices for interpreting big data studies in otolaryngology. We will discuss (1) the rapid expansion of big data research, benefits of large database research, and situations in which big data can help answer important research questions; (2) common pitfalls of studies utilizing large databases; and (3) practical strategies to apply studies using big data to your clinical otolaryngology practice.

Rapid expansion in big data research and areas where big data is most useful

There are a number of factors driving the rapid expansion of otolaryngologic research utilizing big data in recent years (Table 4.1). First, big data studies provide a large sample size, which can increase statistical power and the ability to capture more rare outcomes. Second, big data studies are efficient to conduct—data are already collected, they are usually inexpensive, and participant recruitment is not necessary. Finally, big data studies permit increased external validity and generalizability compared to other study designs.

There are certain clinical questions which are best answered using studies that rely on big data, particularly those from clinical and/or administrative sources. Relative to other potential study designs, big data studies are excellent to: (1) characterize rare diseases (e.g., presentations, outcomes, risk and protective factors, rare diseases or outcomes, and predicting prognosis and staging); (2) evaluate the incidence, prevalence, and impact of certain diagnoses; (3) analyze trends of utilization, cost, and quality care over time; (4) describe sociodemographic factors in relation to areas such as access and outcomes; (5) compare practices in different regions, institutions, specialties, or providers; and (6) evaluate and compare the effectiveness and/or safety of different treatments. Research investigating patient outcomes, risk factors and protective factors, rare diagnoses and outcomes, practice patterns, utilization, and performance can emphasize gaps in delivering quality care and help identify targets for policy, clinical practice guidelines, or quality improvement interventions to enhance the quality and equity of care delivery.[14] Table 4.2 provides examples of different kinds of big data research from across the breadth of otolaryngology (e.g., pediatric otolaryngology, head and neck cancer, rhinology, etc.) utilizing a variety of different big data sources.

Table 4.1 Advantages of big data research.

Advantage	How big data supports this
Large sample size/ statistical power	- Allows for increased power (the likelihood of detecting a statistically significant result when one truly exists).
Efficiency (resources, time, funds)	- Does not require recruiting or following-up with participants. - Data are already collected. - Is often IRB-exempt due to de-identified data, further easing time constraints.[11,12]
Increased external validity of findings	- Allows for increased external validity (the degree that findings can be extrapolated to the target population) due to including a larger, and more representative, population from different regions and institutions.[13]

Table 4.2 Common big data research study designs.

Type of big data study	Analysis features and Clinical utility of findings	Example (year): Data source	Key findings
Evaluate disease characteristics	1. Describe disease phenotypes, presentations, progression patterns, and outcomes (e.g., mortality and survival rates)	Burton et al.[17] (2019): NIS	For patients with invasive fungal rhinosinusitis, underlying immune dysfunction and type of fungal infection (mucormycosis vs. aspergillosis) were associated with early inpatient mortality following ESS.[17]
	2. Describe disease risk and protective factors	Simmonds et al.[18] (2017): KID & NIS	LCH was associated with an increased incidence of chronic OM, OME, chronic sinusitis, and hearing loss. There was no significant association between cholesteatoma and LCH.[18]
	3. Study rare diseases or subgroups of uncommon types of certain diagnoses	Hamdi et al.[19] (2022): VAERS	Among 20 patients with VFP following COVID-19 vaccination, the mean age was 61.8 years and 65% of patients were female. The most common symptom was hoarse voice; most cases were unilateral, and mean time for symptom onset was 12.1 days.[19]
	4. Estimate prognosis and/or staging for certain diagnoses or form predictive models using patient comorbidities to weigh the risks and benefits of different treatments[14–16]	Shay et al.[20] (2022): PHIS	For pediatric patients with bilateral vocal fold dysfunction, gastrointestinal comorbidities and tracheostomy were associated with improved inpatient survival. Tracheostomy was associated with increased cost, comorbidities, gastrostomy tube placement, and a Chiari diagnosis.[20]
Describe epidemiological factors	1. Analyze disease incidence and prevalence	Reid et al.[21] (2021): KID	Estimated incidence of Treacher Collins syndrome was 1 in 80,000. The 3 most common associated diagnoses were gastrostomy, tracheostomy status, and OSA. The most common procedures performed were for airway examination.[21]
	2. Describe impact of certain diseases on the population, such as cost patterns for certain diagnoses and their treatments	McCoul et al.[22] (2019): MarketScan	Over half of patients with ETD were treated with ≥1 prescription medication. Chronic ETD (11% of overall ETD) was most commonly treated with intranasal corticosteroids and antibiotics. Annual cost of prescriptions for ETD was over $8.5 million, with a mean of $80.78 per patients who filled a prescription.[22]
	3. Evaluate how the incidence, prevalence, or severity of a particular disease varies among different subgroups or changes over time	Alexander et al.[23] (2016): VHA EMR	Sleep disorder prevalence increased sixfold from 2000 to 2010. The largest increases were in those with PTSD, other mental health disorders, or combat experience.[23]

Analyze trends in cost, utilization, and quality of care	1. Analyze certain disease or treatment characteristics before and after policy changes	Barnes et al.[24] (2022): SEER	ACA expansion of coverage options for low-income individuals and mandated mental health care coverage was associated with a decrease in suicide incidence for nonelderly patients with cancer, especially young adults in Medicaid expansion versus nonexpansion states.[24]
	2. Describe practice changes before and after policy changes, new or modified guidelines within the field, changes in standard practice, or addition of new practices	Smolinski et al.[25] (2022): MarketScan	Management of uncomplicated, nonrecurrent AOM with guideline-recommended watchful waiting was limited, stagnant across the time period, and driven by clinician factors rather than patient factors.[25]
	3. Form data for future guidelines, correlate changes in outcomes after implementing new practices	Jin et al.[26] (2021): MarketScan	Intratympanic steroids were increasingly used as an adjunctive or alternative to oral steroids for SSNHL management. Repeat intratympanic steroid injections was associated with an increased risk of persistent TM perforations and subsequent tympanoplasty.[26]
Define association of sociodemographic factors with healthcare cost, utilization, and outcomes	1. Explore socioeconomic and demographic factors in relation to healthcare access and resources	Huang et al.[27] (2018): SAS	There were statistical differences in charges, primary payer, household income, and race in children receiving cochlear implantation among four states.[27]
	2. Analyze association of sociodemographic factors (ethnicity, race, gender, sexuality, age, disability status, comorbidities, area of residence, income, insurance coverage) with outcomes	Mullen et al.[28] (2021): NSQIP-P	Racial and ethnic disparities existed in the receipt of primary cleft lip and cleft palate repair, time to repair, and risk of readmission following repair.[28]
Describe practice patterns at the level of providers, institution, or regions	1. Benchmark data and highlight areas for quality improvement in areas like patient demographics, workup and diagnostic procedure guideline adherence, management of similar diagnoses, and outcomes[29]	Adams et al.[31] (2022): OptumLabs Data Warehouse	Use of guideline-discordant neuroimaging for dizziness was prevalent.[31]
	2. Analyze provider factors (e.g., region, department, academic or community institution, hospital RVUs, center size, and resources)[30]	Jang et al.[32] (2021): MarketScan	The most commonly prescribed medication for CRS was antibiotics. Surgery, oral steroids, and antibiotics were most common in the South; Northeast had highest HCE. HCRU and HCE were higher in urban areas.[32]

Continued

Table 4.2 Common big data research study designs.—*cont'd*

Type of big data study	Analysis features and Clinical utility of findings	Example (year): Data source	Key findings
Assess and compare treatments and procedures: cost, risks, benefits	**1.** Evaluate and/or compare different procedures or therapies in regard to risks, benefits, cost-effectiveness, outcomes	Wick et al.[34] (2021): MarketScan	For patients with mandible fractures undergoing surgical repair, prophylactic antibiotic use was not associated with revision surgery, local infection, or osteomyelitis, regardless of repair type.[34]
	2. Utilize data to drive the basis for new techniques or tools for decisionmaking or treatment algorithms	Moroco et al.[35] (2021): NSQIP	For senior patients undergoing transcervical Zenker's diverticulectomy, smoking status was associated with postoperative complications. Age was not an independent risk factor for adverse outcomes.[35]
		Youn et al.[36] (2022): MarketScan	1.1% of patients who received a septoplasty underwent revision. Patients who were older, in the Midwest, or had high-deductible health plans were less likely to undergo revision septoplasty.[36]
		Ibrahim et al.[37] (2021): MarketScan	Soft tissue surgery for adults with OSA was associated with lower rates of cardiovascular, neurological, and endocrine systemic complications compared to CPAP prescription.[37]

ACA, Affordable Care Act; AOM, Acute otitis media; CPAP, Continuous Positive Airway Pressure; EMR, Electronic medical record; ETD, Eustachian tube dysfunction; HCE, Healthcare expenditure; HCRU, Healthcare resource utilization; HCUP, Healthcare Cost and Utilization Project; KID, Kids' Inpatient Database (by HCUP); LCH, Langerhans Cell Histiocytosis; NSQIP, American College of Surgeons National Surgical Quality Improvement Program; NSQIP-P, NSQIP Pediatric; OM, Otitis media; OME, Otitis media with effusion; OSA, Obstructive sleep apnea; PHIS, Pediatric Health Information System; PTSD, Posttraumatic stress disorder; RVU, Relative value units; SAS, HCUP State Ambulatory surgery services database (of California, Florida, Maryland, New York, Kentucky); SEER, Surveillance, Epidemiology, and End Results Program; SSNHL, sudden sensorineural hearing loss; TM, Tympanic membrane; VAERS, Vaccine Adverse Event Reporting System database; VFP, Vocal fold paresis or paralysis; VHA, US Veterans Health Administration.

Common pitfalls in big data studies

We will now discuss pitfalls within big data studies, which exist in three overarching (although at times overlapping) categories: (1) Pitfalls in study design; (2) pitfalls in data analysis; and (3) pitfalls of interpreting study findings.

Common pitfalls in big data study design (study sample, setting, participants)—Selection bias, observation bias, and missing data

When considering the design of a big data study, important pitfalls include selection bias (both of patients included in the database and in the study cohort formed from the database), observation bias, and missing data. Each of these considerations is important because they can introduce bias. Bias is a systematic error in estimations of "truth," the conceptual equivalent of being off to the left of the "target." Bias results in incorrect and/or invalid estimates of "truth." Although bias is a threat to all research study designs, it is particularly relevant to consider when reading big data literature. Each is discussed below with relevant examples from the otolaryngologic literature.

Selection bias of patients included in the database

Selection bias refers to systematic differences in the characteristics of patients included in the study sample relative to patients in the target population. Most databases sample patients based on specific methods (e.g., region of the US, health insurance coverage, diagnosis, treatment type, treatment facility type). As a result, the database generally does not include all of the patients in the target patient population. Selection bias may therefore arise if patients included in the database systematically differ from the target population. Table 4.3 summarizes instances of selection bias of patients included in big data studies.

Selection bias also affects big data studies that utilize the EHR. EHR-based big data studies are generally limited to a single health system or institution and thus findings may not be as generalizable to different regions or populations. For example, patients treated at Veterans Health Administration (VHA) and its integrated EMR allow for national evaluations. However, veterans are older and more often identify as male and non-Hispanic white compared to the US population.[41]

Selection bias within data sets (deriving a study cohort)

In addition to selection bias that may arise from the choice of a database, an additional layer of selection bias may occur during the application of specific inclusion and exclusion criteria to form the study cohort from the database. To include all patients who received different therapies for a certain diagnosis in a given time period and/or region, investigators must identify the International Classification of Diseases (ICD) codes associated with that diagnosis and the Current Procedural Terminology

Table 4.3 Selection bias of patients included in big data.

Big data example	Patients included	How sampling method may affect big data studies
Sampling by health insurance coverage		
MarketScan Commercial and Medicare Databases	Administrative claim-based sampling. Both databases only include patients with some form of employer-based health insurance	Overrepresentation of patients with employer-based insurance and underrepresentation of those with public insurance relative to the general US population.[38]
MarketScan Multistate Medicaid Database	Medicaid-enrolled patients in 11 states	Medicaid enrollees tend to be of lower socioeconomic status compared to the national US population, so findings using this database may not be as generalizable to patients with other payment methods.[1]
SEER	Population-based database (sampling patients to mimic the general US population), representing about 48% of the US population including clinical, demographic, and cause of death information for patients with cancer.[39]	SEER and Medicare claims data are often linked (SEER-Medicare), which allows a more comprehensive view of the continuum of care before, during, and following cancer diagnosis and treatment. However, patients who are Medicare beneficiaries tend to be older than the general US population, so findings may not be as generalizable to younger patients.
Medicare claims data	Collects information from the time of patients' Medicare eligibility until death	
Sampling based on facility types		
NCDB	Patients treated at facilities accredited by the CoC[1]	Systematic differences could exist between patients treated at CoC-accredited facilities and those treated at non-CoC facilities (e.g., cancer stage, insurance status) or care processes at Coc-accredited and nonaccredited facilities (e.g., adherence to guidelines, clinical volume, more accessible resources).
NSQIP	Random sample of patients treated at > 700 participating hospitals	Data may systematically underrepresent rare procedures, disease processes, and outcomes. Data may overrepresent large academic hospitals with more funding and quality accreditations.[14,40]
	Primarily samples patients undergoing general, vascular, and multispecialty surgeries and excludes minor procedures (which are common in otolaryngology)	Cases within otolaryngology can be underrepresented; Tang et al. found that <40% of otolaryngologic procedure cases were represented (as opposed to about 99.7% for vascular surgery).[13]

Table 4.3 Selection bias of patients included in big data.—*cont'd*

Big data example	Patients included	How sampling method may affect big data studies
Sampling by care delivery setting (inpatient, ambulatory surgery, ED)		
NIS	Inclusion of patients of all payer type who undergo inpatient surgery	For any procedure that can be performed in the ambulatory or inpatient setting (e.g., cochlear implant, thyroidectomy), selection bias can ensue. Patients who are treated inpatient may systematically differ than those treated in outpatient (age, comorbidity, complex anatomical features, frailty, risk of adverse outcomes).
SASD	Ambulatory procedures and other outpatient services from hospital-owned (and some free-standing) ambulatory facilities in 35 participating states, including patients from all payer types	

CoC, *Commission on Cancer;* ED, *Emergency Department;* NCDB, *National Cancer Database;* NIS, *National Inpatient Sample;* NSQIP, *American College of Surgeons National Surgical Quality Improvement Program;* SASD, *State Ambulatory Surgery and Services Database;* SEER, *Surveillance, Epidemiology, and End Results Program.*

(CPT) codes that capture the procedures of interest. Any variations or errors in methods to form the study cohort allow for different patient samples to be extracted from the same database and included in the study cohorts, as demonstrated in the retrieval bag surgical site infection analyses.[2,8,9]

A study by Bur et al. showed how application of specific study eligibility criteria can result in very different study findings.[42] The researchers were interested in whether there was an association between surgical specialty (plastic surgery or otolaryngology) and clinical outcomes for patients who underwent microvascular head and neck reconstruction.[43] The eligibility criteria for cohort 1 included all free tissue reconstruction procedures performed by one of the two specialties from 2005 to 2018 (2072 plastic surgery cases; 3313 otolaryngology cases). In cohort 2, authors used the same eligibility criteria with an additional inclusion criterion of a head and neck malignancy diagnosis (by ICD codes) or ablative head and neck surgery (CPT codes) during the same operation. The additional criterion resulted in the exclusion of 1493 (72.1%) cases performed by plastic surgeons and 286 (8.6%) cases performed by otolaryngologists. Analyses from cohort 1 (including patients with reconstructive surgery not limited to the head and neck) showed otolaryngology cases to have higher complication rates and longer LOS than plastic surgery, but cohort 2 (only including patients with head and neck reconstruction) found plastic surgery cases to have more complications and longer LOS. The patients in cohort 1 who were treated by otolaryngologists were older, had more severe comorbidities, and were more malnourished compared to the patients treated by plastic surgeons, which might be expected because most patients in the plastic surgery arm of cohort 1 did not represent the target population of patients with head and neck cancer. This study displayed how variation in study cohort derivation can introduce selection bias and drastically alter findings. Additionally, it highlighted how big data can facilitate exploring all types of questions, even those in which findings might not add significant value to patient care, and could even contribute to strain in professional communities.[42]

Observation bias

Another potential pitfall of big data research is observation bias, or error arising from systematic differences in either the way information about exposure or disease is obtained from the study groups. For example, patients with certain characteristics, such as lack of transportation or residence being further from the institution, may be less likely to return to the institution where data are gathered for information about outcomes of interest (e.g., survival, patterns of recurrence), leading to observed differences in outcomes. If patients of a certain population fail to return to an institution due to distance from the facility or lack of transportation, researchers might never know if those patients were readmitted or experienced other adverse outcomes. While this type of bias affects all observational study designs, the potential for observation bias may be larger in big database studies because the way data are collected does not allow researchers to know why specific patients received certain treatments or procedures over alternative approaches. For example, Graboyes et al. conducted an NCDB analysis to evaluate the effect of postoperative radiation (PORT) delays on survival in patients with head and neck squamous cell carcinoma (HNSCC). Researchers found that PORT delays were associated with decreased survival. However, observational bias may affect the findings of this study, with the authors noting the inability to discern specific reasons of why patients experienced delays. Possible underlying explanations for delays include tumor board discussions, collaboration with patients and providers concerning the risks and benefits of PORT, referral and scheduling processes to begin PORT on time, patient and family preferences, patient hesitancy or indecisiveness, access to care, and ability to take time off from daily obligations to attend appointments.[44]

Missing data

Big data studies are affected by missing data, which are generally neither uniform nor missing at random and thus have the potential to bias study findings. One example of missing data is when certain individual patients have missing values for particular variables or outcomes within a database. In addition to data fields that are present within the database for which select patients may have missing values, databases are also limited in which data fields they collect. Each database varies in terms of what variables it collects based on the primary purpose of the database (e.g., administrative, billing, quality improvement, or clinical research). Finally, databases may have nuanced specific to ways in which data are captured/coded. These three ways that missing data may affect big data studies are illustrated in Table 4.4.

Table 4.4 Missing data.

Data source	Examples of missing data and how it affects big data research	Illustration in the literature
Missing data values for individual patients		
NSQIP	Patients can have missing laboratory values, vital status, comorbidities, functional outcomes, complications, and more. These missing data can cause difficulty in ascertaining the effect of laboratory values or preexisting conditions on operative outcomes.	Patients undergoing cancer resection who were less healthy and undergoing more risky procedures were more likely to have complete laboratory values and fewer missing data reported. The ability of some variables (e.g., white blood cell count, PTT, and significant weight loss) to predict major complications significantly changed when patients with missing data were removed.[45]
ARIC	Patients with factors that impair their ability to complete certain testing (such as cognitive testing) could be excluded from analyses, which could lead to under- or overestimation of associations. For example, failure to complete cognitive testing could be due to inability to hear auditory testing stimuli, fatigue, and education attainment.	Researchers hypothesized that missing data were contributing to underestimating the association between HI and cognitive decline and conducted an analysis to compare the likelihood of completing cognitive testing in older adults with HI versus those without HI. The authors reported that patients with HI were less likely to complete cognitive testing, contributing to missing data for cognitive variables. Simply disregarding missing data underestimated the correlation between HI and cognition by 30%.[46]
Missing data by what variables are collected in the data source		
NSQIP	Collects data for only 30 days following surgery. Therefore, long-term safety, functional, and/or QOL outcomes cannot be studied.[42,47]	Cochlear implant outcomes study cited the limitation of being unable to evaluate AOM because the median time to presentation following implant is 6 months.[48]
	Because NSQIP is intended primarily for general surgery, it does not include some variables that are particularly important to otolaryngologists. This leads to the inability to ascertain certain outcomes (e.g., tracheostomy or gastrostomy dependence, preoperative radiation or chemotherapy) or outcomes themselves (e.g., peripheral nerve injury, disease recurrence, or graft failure).[42,49–52]	In a study to analyze factors associated with CSF leak following skull base surgery, authors noted that many variables potentially associated with risk of CSF leak (e.g., tumor size and characteristics, histopathology, resection extent, and disease laterality) are not captured in NSQIP and thus could not be analyzed as part of the study.[53]

Continued

Table 4.4 Missing data.—*cont'd*

Data source	Examples of missing data and how it affects big data research	Illustration in the literature
NCDB	Reports vital status (alive, not alive) at last follow-up, but does not gather data regarding cause of death, functional outcomes, or patient-reported outcomes like QOL. Additional variables that can affect outcomes (smoking status, alcohol use) are not collected.	Researchers comparing TORS to nonsurgical treatment for HPV-negative OPSCC noted that the evaluation of oncologic outcomes was restricted to overall survival because disease recurrence and cause of death are not included in the NCDB. Additionally, the authors stated that functional outcomes are essential in both treatment decision-making and assessing oncologic outcomes, and the inability to assess them is a limitation of the findings.[54]
NIS	Does not report mortality and complications following discharge. Factors that can influence access to care, including baseline health status, education attainment, and employment status, are not collected.	In an analysis to identify racial disparities in charges, LOS, and complications for adults receiving inpatient epistaxis treatment, researchers stated that the lack of collecting mortality and complications likely results in underreporting of postoperative adverse outcomes. Authors also highlighted the limited ability to account for potential confounding factors that affect access to care and outcomes. Epistaxis site and episode severity were unable to be evaluated.[55]
Nuanced specific ways in which data are captured/coded		
NCDB	Reports readmission within 30 days of surgery, but only includes readmissions to the original institution where the index surgery occurred.	Studies have estimated that this coding omits an estimated 12% −33% of postoperative readmissions, therefore underestimating readmission rates for patients.[11,56–59]

AOM, *Acute otitis media;* ARIC, *Atherosclerosis Risk in Communities;* CSF, *Cerebrospinal fluid;* HI, *Hearing impairment;* HPV, *Human Papillomavirus;* LOS, *Length of stay;* NCDB, *National Cancer Database;* NIS, *National Inpatient Sample;* NSQIP, *National Surgical Quality Improvement Program;* OPSCC, *Oropharyngeal Squamous Cell Carcinoma;* QOL, *Quality of life;* TORS, *Transoral Robotic Surgery.*

Common pitfalls in big data analysis—Confounding and immortal time bias

After considering potential pitfalls in the big data study design, it is critical to evaluate common pitfalls in the data analysis.

Confounding

One important pitfall that is common in the analysis of big data is confounding. Confounding occurs when an apparent association between the independent variable (exposure) and dependent variable (outcome) is actually caused by a third variable that is related to both the exposure and outcome. In some situations, the confounding variable is known and can be controlled for during the analysis. In other situations, the confounding variable is not known and thus cannot be controlled for during the analysis. Confounding and missing data are conceptually distinct but closely related in large database studies.

Confounding is a consideration for all observational studies, not just those using secondary datasets. Confounding variables that are not included into databases, or not included wholly, can cause an inaccurate estimate of the size of an apparent association between an exposure and outcome.[60] This is a common effect observed when factors that affect treatment decisions are also determinants of outcomes, such as in poor baseline health status.[61] Factors including a patient's baseline health status, disease prognosis, patient and clinician past experiences with the particular treatment, and the patient's capability and willingness to undergo a particular therapy or procedure can affect the likelihood that a certain patient gets a particular treatment.[62] This was illustrated in a study by Cole et al. evaluating the association of patient age and frailty with postoperative outcomes in adults following cochlear implantation (CI) using data from the NIS. In this study, the authors found no association between frailty and postoperative complications. However, in the limitations, the authors pointed out that the lack of association between frailty and postoperative complications could potentially be explained by selection bias: patients who were audiologic candidates for CI but considered too frail for surgery may never receive a CI. Therefore, studying the link between outcomes of CI and frailty is challenging using the NIS as only patients healthy enough (with lower complication risk) to undergo CI surgery will be included, and the potential association between complication rates and age and frailty is likely undermined.[63]

The best way to control for confounding in the design phase is to randomly allocate patients to study arms. However, this is not possible in secondary datasets. Minimizing bias due to confounding in these situations requires controlling for confounding variables through statistical analytic tools such as multivariable regression analysis. Unfortunately, statistical methods to minimize confounding can only be applied to measured variables (i.e., cannot be applied to variables that are missing), and the success of the analytic technique depends in part on the accuracy of the coding of the potential confounding variable.[62] Confounding variables that are not accounted for can cause unmeasured or residual confounding.[11,29]

The interaction between missing data and unmeasured confounding variables was illustrated in the previously mentioned NSQIP study by Perry et al. analyzing factors associated with CSF leak following skull base surgery.[53] In the study, Perry et al. used NSQIP data to analyze factors associated with cerebrospinal fluid (CSF) leak following skull base surgery for schwannoma, meningioma, pituitary tumor, or trigeminal neuralgia. The authors found that lumbar drain placement and skull base reconstruction were both associated with higher rates of CSF leak. However, prior studies suggested that they were associated with *lower* CSF leak rates.[64-66] The unexpected finding that lumbar drain placement and skull base reconstruction increased the risk of CSF leak could potentially be explained by a number of confounding variables related to the extent of surgery (e.g., larger tumor size, tumors requiring more bony removal for exposure, intraoperative complications).[53] In this example, the extent of the surgery likely confounds the relationship between lumbar drain placement and postoperative CSF leak, as extensive surgeries are associated with both lumbar drain placement and the risk of postoperative CSF leak. Since variables describing the extent of surgery are not included in NSQIP, there is an unmeasured potential confounding variable for the relationship between lumbar drain and postoperative CSF leak in this study.[53]

Immortal time bias

A specific form of confounding, known as immortal time bias, is also frequently encountered in big data studies. Immortal time bias can occur when there is a period of follow-up during which the outcome of interest cannot occur. For example, patients cannot experience a hospital readmission if they have yet to be discharged from the primary admission, making them "immortal" to readmission until initial discharge. When studying hospital readmission rates, patients with an LOS over 30 days after surgery cannot have the outcome of interest (i.e., readmission within 30 days of surgery). NSQIP, and any other database that tracks patient outcomes up to 30 days postoperatively rather than 30 days following hospital discharge, is susceptible to immortal time bias for readmission.

The potential for immortal time bias was highlighted in a study by Lucas et al. using NSQIP to analyze the frequency of postoperative readmission for patients undergoing various surgical subspecialty operations. Lucas et al. observed that readmission rates increased with prolonged LOS, peaked at an LOS of 13 days, and then decreased for LOS > 13 days.[67] The authors conducted additional analyses to investigate the effects of immortal time bias on the apparent rate of postoperative hospital readmissions within 30 days of discharge in NSQIP. The researchers included patients at a single institution who were captured in NSQIP and compared EMR-obtained readmission (up to 30-days following *discharge*) to NSQIP (30-days after *surgery*) readmission rates. Of 707 patients included, 134 (18.9%) experienced a readmission; of those, 114 (16.1%) were readmitted within 30 days postoperatively and 20 (2.8%) were readmitted >30 days postoperatively. Patients with an LOS over 25 days had low readmission rates in NSQIP (i.e., within 30-days of surgery), likely because of concealed data (the patients with LOS > 25 days were less likely to be readmitted within the 5 days remaining that NSQIP would capture readmission). The authors stated that if immortal time bias is not accounted for, patients with longer postoperative LOS (and likely more postoperative complications and morbidity) appear to have low readmission rates in NSQIP.[68] In summary, due to immortal time bias, NSQIP analyses tend to underestimate readmission rates within 30-days of hospital discharge, with worsened bias as LOS lengthens.[67,68]

Common pitfalls of interpreting big data study findings (clinical vs. statistical significance)

A final important pitfall in big data studies involves differentiating statistical versus clinical significance. Statistical significance is established by a predetermined P-value (usually $<.05$ by convention), reflecting the likelihood—5% or less—that differences between groups are due to chance. Conversely, clinical significance is established by the clinician, patient, and/or other relevant stakeholders, and reflects the value of a study outcome that will change management or prognosis. All other things being equal, as the sample size increases, so does likelihood of the findings being statistically significant. Therefore, in big data studies, large sample sizes can allow researchers to identify small differences between groups that are statistically significant (i.e., below the preestablished P-value of statistical significance) but not clinically significant (i.e., the difference is so small that it would not change patient care). When reading articles using big data, it is imperative for the clinicians to decide if statistically significant findings are also clinically significant.

With a large enough sample size or high enough measurement precision, a minute effect can accompany a significant P-value.[69] For example, Kou et al. sought to analyze if pediatric tonsillectomy outcomes were affected by mental health disorders using KID and the Nationwide Readmission Database (NRD). The study included 37,386 children who had a tonsillectomy, 2138 of which were diagnosed with a mental health disorder. The mean age of patients who had mental health disorders was 6.0 years, while the mean of the patients without a mental health disorder was 5.3 years. This difference of 0.7 years was statistically significant ($P < .001$), likely partially due to the large patient sample.[70] Conversely, Favre et al. conducted a study using KID to analyze incidence and management of acute mastoiditis-related complications in children. The mean age difference of 0.74 years between the 80 patients with intracranial abscess (7.73 years) and the 1981 patients without intracranial abscess (6.99 years) was not statistically significant ($P = .183$).[71]

Additionally, relying solely on the statistically significance of results to deduce clinical importance of a study allows researchers and clinicians to overlook important differences that did not reach a P-value below the cutoff or assume that all statistically significant results will impact patients and their care.[72] Piccirillo et al. utilized big data to evaluate success rates of first-line antibiotics versus new, costlier second-line medications in treating uncomplicated sinusitis.[73] There was a 90.1% treatment success rate for the 17,329 patients who received first-line antibiotics, while the 11,773 who received second-line antibiotics had a 90.8% success rate; a statistically significant difference of 0.7% (95%CI 0.0%–1.4%, $P < .05$). However, the authors noted that the absolute difference in success between groups treated with first-line versus more expensive second-line antibiotics was actually small and clinically insignificant.[73]

While *P*-values place focus on data being dichotomized into either "significance" or "insignificance" based on an arbitrary cutoff, confidence intervals (CIs) represent the estimates more completely, aiding in discerning clinical and statistical significance and further allowing for interpreting clinical relevance.[69,74] Consider a patient education intervention to lower postoperative readmissions, where researchers predetermine a 10% or greater decrease in readmission rates from baseline to be clinically significant.[69] If the results revealed a 7% decrease in readmission ($P = .08$, 95%CI -1%−15%), solely interpreting based on *P*-value would represent a statistically insignificant decrease in readmission. However, the upper bound of CI suggests that the intervention was associated with up to 15% lesser readmissions, and the lower bound suggests that the program could be associated with either no change (CI includes 0) or a 1% *increase* in readmissions. These results are inconclusive, but merit further investigation because of the possibility that the intervention was associated with up to 15% lesser readmissions. The *P*-value alone represents statistically insignificant results in this study and an ineffective intervention, which is an incorrect conclusion based on further inspection of CIs.[69]

In summary, statistical and clinical significance are both important, but not equivalent. A threshold should be established for clinical significance. CIs and *P*-values can be seen as two sides of a coin, with *P*-values providing statistical significance and evidence against likelihood of false positives and CIs including a range of possible values for the effect size estimate, which can be used to determine statistical significance and clinical relevance.[75]

Steps to incorporating big data research into your clinical practice

Taking a systematic approach to medical literature will help with understanding the study findings and relating them to the otolaryngologist's practice and patient population. There are three overarching steps, which include (1) engaging the literature with purpose; (2) identifying study objectives; and (3) recognizing common pitfalls in large database research.

Engage the biomedical literature with a specific purpose (decide how to interact)

Evidence-based medicine incorporates the best available evidence with a practitioner's knowledge to answer clinical inquiries.[76] Staying updated on the large amount of biomedical literature published daily can be demanding. Moreover, it is impossible to apply the scrutiny outlined in this chapter to each article that is encountered. Therefore, a critical step to approaching biomedical literature is to engage with a specific purpose. There are different strategies to interact with articles in the literature, which vary based on how relevant a given article is to one's practice or interests. Neely et al. proposed the "Quick scan/rapid read/study" method to approaching literature. The "Quick Scan" consists of scanning titles of articles in a journal's table of contents and marking those one might be interested in. This step is just so that one is aware of what new evidence has been published. The "Rapid Read" involves reading abstract conclusions in the articles that were marked, which can eventually be combined with the first step. Third is the "Read Completely" step, where the authors suggest choosing one or two articles to read fully. Lastly, the "Study" phase comprises critically engaging with and analyzing the article in its entirety, maybe even suggesting its discussion in a journal club or other setting. This final step is where one may encounter practice-changing findings.[76]

Understand the objective(s) of the study

The second imperative step in incorporating big data literature into clinical practice is understanding what category the objective(s) of a study fall into. Understanding the objectives will help with recognizing the importance or applicability of the findings to patients. As shown in Table 4.5, common objectives utilized in big data analyses include descriptive, hypothesis-generating, and hypothesis-testing.

Identify sources of bias to evaluate the internal validity of the study

Otolaryngologists who read big data studies my apply findings to inform and improve their clinical practice. However, as described in detail in Understand the objective(s) of the study, big data studies have numerous potential pitfalls that can undermine the validity of study findings. Being aware of the possible shortcomings of research using big data can help lessen problems with interpreting findings, advance the validity of findings, and allow for the translation of analyses into clinical practice.[79] Here we will provide practical advice to help the otolaryngologist mitigate potential pitfalls of big data research.

Addressing pitfalls in study design—Selection bias, observation bias, and missing data

i. **Selection bias:** To mitigate sample bias that may result from the specific eligibility criteria used in the big data study, readers should carefully review study inclusion and exclusion criteria. This information is often presented in the methods section of manuscripts and may include the specific diagnosis and treatment codes utilized, along with how the reliability was verified. For example, Ho et al. sought to evaluate the independent impact of total number of positive lymph nodes (LNs) on survival in oral cavity squamous cell carcinoma (OCSCC) using data from the NCDB. The researchers included adults with primary OCSCC treated from 2004 to 2013 with upfront surgical resection for curative intent and neck dissection with at least 10 LNs. Patients included in the NCDB who were diagnosed with squamous cell neoplasms were identified

Table 4.5 Big data research objectives.

Objective type	Description, key points, and use	Example (year): Data source	Example (objective)	Example (results and conclusions)
Descriptive	- Describe occurrences in a certain population in the form of trends or relationships - Provide general descriptions about practices - May include data about prognoses, disease incidence, and patterns of care delivery - Do *not* use inferential statistics (making assumptions about the "truth" in a target population)	Chung et al.[15] (2017): SEER	" … to *investigate the epidemiology, tumor characteristics, and survival of PedsSNM* using a population-based database to augment the scant literature on this topic."[15]	Reported demographics, incidence, most frequent malignancy and primary site, tumor grades, disease-specific survival rates, and factors associated with survival in patients with PedsSNM.
Hypothesis-generating	- Evaluate differences between groups or primary outcomes to generate a hypothesis. - Conclusions may include phrases like "future studies are needed to … " - Formed hypothesis will be the basis for another study that will be more confirmatory, utilizing inferential statistics.	Rudmik et al.[77] (2017): DIMR	" … to *evaluate differences* in surgeon-specific performance for ESS using a risk-adjusted 5-year ESS revision rate as a quality metric … primary outcomes."[77]	Conclusion: " … *future studies are needed to evaluate* more surgeon-specific variables and validate a risk adjustment model to provide appropriate feedback for quality improvement."

Table 4.5 Big data research objectives.—*cont'd*

Objective type	Description, key points, and use	Example (year): Data source	Example (objective)	Example (results and conclusions)
Hypothesis-testing	- Will test a hypothesis that might be specific differences (outcomes, survival) between two treatment groups or populations - May inquire if patients treated with one modality have better outcomes or survival, although these participants *are not randomized.* - Implement inferential statistics to test the formed hypothesis and make inferences about "truth" in target population	Zumsteg et al.[78] (2017): NCDB	" … *hypothesized* that aggressive treatment of primary tumor site would be associated with improved survival for patients with metastatic HNSCC receiving chemotherapy."[78]	Conclusion: "Aggressive local treatment *warrants prospective evaluation* for select patients with metastatic HNSCC."

DIMR, *Data Integration, Measurement, and Reporting Administrative Database;* ESS, *Endoscopic sinus surgery;* HNSCC, *Head and Neck Squamous Cell Carcinoma;* NCDB, *National Cancer Database;* PedsSNM, *Pediatric sinonasal malignancies;* SEER, *Surveillance, Epidemiology, and End Results Program.*

using International Classification of Diseases for Oncology, third edition (ICD-O-3) codes 8050–8084. Additionally, Table 4.6 depicts the ICD-O-3 codes. Ho et al. used to select patients with specific OCSCC subtypes and exclude patients with ambiguous or overlapping sites that could be oropharyngeal origin.[80] To further inform readers about the validity of data, any routine quality checks that are performed on the database as well as previous research completed utilizing the database should be cited.[81] Often big data studies will include flow diagrams that display the stepwise process of initial case identification and the application of specific inclusion and exclusion criterion. These diagrams help a reader to understand which type/why certain patients were included/excluded

Table 4.6 ICD-O-3 codes used as inclusion and exclusion criteria for patients with specific cancer subtypes.

Specific subtypes included	ICD-O-3 codes
Oral tongue	C02.0-C02.3
Upper/lower gum	C03.0-C03.9
Floor of mouth	C04.0-C04.9
Hard palate	C05.0
Other parts of mouth (e.g., buccal mucosa, retromolar trigone)	C06.0-C06.9
Exclusion criteria—sites that could be oropharyngeal origin	**ICD-O-3 codes**
Tongue/base of tongue	C02.8-C02.9
Hard palate/soft palate	C05.8-C05.9

Based on Ho AS, Kim S, Tighiouart M, et al. Metastatic lymph node burden and survival in oral cavity cancer. J Clin Oncol 2017;35(31):3601−3609.

and also the magnitude of eligibility criteria on the study sample. When implemented correctly, flow diagrams should allow another researcher to replicate the study and arrive at the same conclusions.[11] Fig. 4.1 depicts the flow diagram of study cohort derivation from Goel et al., who utilized the NCDB to evaluate the impact of treatment package time on survival in patients with surgically treated HNSCC followed by PORT.[82] By analyzing the flow diagram, readers can see how researchers reduced the original sample of 395,821 to the final study cohort including 35,167 patients who met eligibility criteria.

ii. **Missing data:** When reading a big data study, otolaryngologists should pay specific attention to missing data. This may include data that are missing because the variables are not captured in the database or data missing for individual patients for whom the included variable was not measured. Often authors will detail methods to address missing data and why a particular method was chosen over alternatives. Readers should look for these types of statements. Often this will include phrases like "values were imputed …" as well as rationale for exclusion criteria.

Additionally, readers should observe tables and figures for missing data, where authors should note the number of patients who did not have a given variable reported. For example, Graboyes et al. sought to evaluate procedure, patient-, and hospital-level risk factors associated with 30-day readmission following inpatient otolaryngologic surgery. The authors utilized the State Inpatient Database (SID) from California. The authors reported that 7.1% of total patients were missing data about race and 1.7% were missing data required to determine median household income (Table 4.7).[83] Noting the missing data as a percentage of the given variable represents one model of presenting missing data. Instead of presenting missing data as a category within a variable, another strategy to be

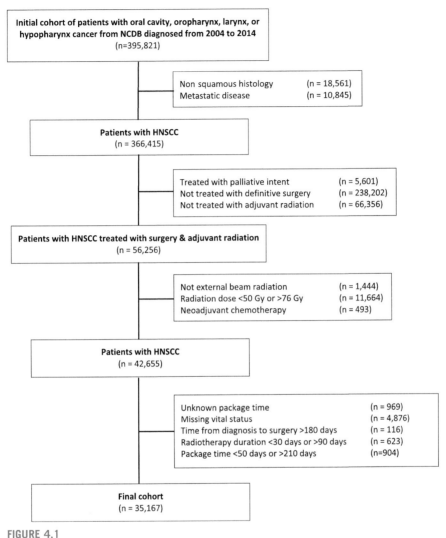

FIGURE 4.1

Flow diagram of study cohort derivation.

Modified from Goel AN, Frangos MI, Raghavan G, et al. The impact of treatment package time on survival in surgically managed head and neck cancer in the United States. Oral Oncol. 2019;88(2019):39—49.

transparent about missing data involves adding superscripts within the variables that refer to a note below the table that displays the number of missing data points for each variable. In all situations, summing the overall N and percentages within a given category allows the reader to check the completeness of data and assess for potential missingness.

Table 4.7 Patient demographics.

Variable		Total Patients (n=58231)	Patients without Readmission (n=53522)	Patients with Readmission (n=4709)
		n (%)	n (%)	n (%)
Race				
	White	33536 (57.6)	30833 (57.6)	2703 (57.4)
	Black	4449 (7.6)	4001 (7.5)	448 (9.5)
	Hispanic	10840 (18.6)	9866 (18.4)	974 (20.7)
	Asian	4204 (7.2)	3844 (7.2)	360 (7.6)
	Other	1064 (1.8)	979 (1.8)	85 (1.8)
	Missing	4138 (7.1)	3999 (7.5)	139 (3.0)
Median household income of ZIP (quartiles)				
	4 (lowest)	12801 (22.0)	11642 (21.8)	1159 (24.6)
	3	14081 (24.2)	12932 (24.2)	1149 (24.4)
	2	14741 (25.3)	13559 (25.3)	1182 (25.1)
	1 (highest)	15603 (26.8)	14464 (27.0)	1139 (24.2)
	Missing	1005 (1.7)	925 (1.7)	80 (1.7)
Insurance				
	Private	28499 (48.9)	26763 (50.0)	1736 (36.9)
	Medicaid	5868 (10.1)	5167 (9.7)	701 (14.9)
	Medicare	16866 (29.0)	14945 (27.9)	1921 (40.8)
	Self-pay	2781 (4.8)	2657 (5.0)	124 (2.6)
	Other	4217 (7.2)	3990 (7.5)	227 (4.8)

Modified from Graboyes EM, Kallogjeri D, Saeed MJ, et al. 30-day hospital readmission following otolaryngology surgery: analysis of a state inpatient database. Laryngoscope, 2017;127(2):337–345.

Addressing pitfalls in data analysis—Confounding and immortal time bias

i. **Confounding:** Researchers may minimize confounding via a variety of statistical adjustments including stratification, multivariable linear or logistic regression analysis, and propensity score matching. Stratification involves creating subgroups based on potential confounding variables (e.g., age, sex, disease severity) and evaluating the association in those different groups to assess whether that variable is confounding the results. Multivariable logistic and linear regression analyses allow researchers to identify independent factors that could affect outcomes. These analyses are similar to stratification, but adjust for multiple, rather than a single confounding variable. The process of propensity score matching attempts to mirror the process of randomization by creating groups with similar possible confounding demographic and/or clinical variables.[29,84,85] Unfortunately, missing data contribute to problems with confounding in big data studies because variables that researchers wish account for may not all be included in a given database. Because not all confounding variables may be accounted for, there is a residual risk of confounding in these analyses that readers should be aware of.

When reading a big data study, otolaryngologists should be mindful of how researchers addressed potential confounding variables. Often researchers will explicitly state the methods that they utilize. For example, Quimby et al. used NSQIP-P to study risk factors for SSIs among pediatric patients undergoing CI. They found that operative duration was associated with significantly increased risk of SSI. They subsequently controlled for a number of potential confounding variables using multivariable logistic regression analysis. To confirm that longer surgical duration was independently associated with an increased risk of SSI, the authors also adjusted for potential confounding variables which might be related to prolonged operative time such as simultaneous bilateral implantation; however, prolonged operative time remained independently associated with an increased risk of SSI on adjusted analyses.[48]

In addition, readers should note the potential for unmeasured residual confounding in the limitations section. Rigorous researchers should include an explicit statement of unmeasured potential confounding variables. Quimby et al. noted unmeasured variables that could be related to longer operation but were likely not related to increased SSI risk, such as differing techniques between surgeons and anatomic abnormalities causing difficult surgery. Further, the authors mentioned different levels of surgeon experience and involvement of trainees as unmeasured potential confounding variables.[48] Moreover, Yan et al. conducted a study using data from the NCDB to evaluate the prognostic role of microscopic extranodal extension and to determine if the addition of chemotherapy concurrent with adjuvant radiotherapy (CRT) improved overall survival (OS) compared to adjuvant radiation therapy (RT) in HPV-negative HNSCC.[86] The authors found that concurrent CRT was not associated with improved OS compared to RT, but noted that unmeasured confounding variables that are strongly related to oncologic outcomes (e.g., specific intensity-modulated RT fields and inadequate chemotherapy dosing) were likely contributing to systematic differences between the two treatment groups and to finding a lack of OS benefit with CRT.[86–89]

ii. **Immortal time bias:** Otolaryngologists reading articles using big data should remain vigilant for the potential for immortal time bias. Often researchers will recognize the bias in the limitations section, state how the findings might be affected, and any methods used to address the bias. Additionally, readers should review the study eligibility criteria for any potential opportunities for immortal time bias and note follow-up period and how the findings might be affected by the bias. To account for immortal time bias in NSQIP analyses, researchers should utilize readmission date, for which NSQIP began reporting in 2012.[68] As an example of addressing this bias, Ho et al. conducted an NCDB and SEER analysis to evaluate the prognostic impact of histologic grade for papillary thyroid carcinoma. Based on recommendations to start adjuvant therapy within

3 months, the researchers performed landmark analysis to exclude patients who died before being able to receive postoperative RT.[90]

Ways to address pitfalls in interpreting big data study findings (statistical vs. clinical significance and clinical significance threshold)

Researchers should acknowledge statistical and clinical significance and provide a reasonable explanation of how a certain cutoff for clinical significance was selected. Readers should ponder what the results actually mean, and if they are clinically meaningful.

Best et al. used NSQIP to compare the use of conventional cautery and alternative energy devices in thyroid surgery outcomes. In the study of 13,330 patients, alternative cautery sources were associated with prolonged operative time by 4.95 min ($P < .0001$). However, the researchers pointed to the fact that this small reduction in operative time might not be clinically significant, and noted that cost-effectiveness of different approaches should be addressed in future publications.[91]

In the previously mentioned Kou et al. study evaluating tonsillectomy outcomes, patients who were diagnosed with a mental health disorder experienced a longer mean LOS (3.4 days) than children without a mental health diagnosis (2.3 days). This mean difference of 1.1 days in the hospital is both statistically significant ($P < .001$) and clinically significant.[70] On the other hand, Etchill et al. utilized NSQIP-P to evaluate outcomes in neonates undergoing thorascopic (n = 133, mean LOS 25 days) versus open repair (n = 722, mean LOS 28 days) for esophageal atresia and tracheoesophageal fistula ($P = .14$).[92] Although the mean difference in LOS between these two groups is not statistically significant, a difference of 3 days admitted to the hospital would be considered by many to be clinically important.

Further, several societies have created tools to assist clinicians interpret findings and ascertain a clinical benefit from statistical findings, like the American Society of Clinical Oncology's (ASCO's) Value Framework and the European Society for Medical Oncology's (ESMO's) Magnitude of Clinical Benefit Scale created to interpret cancer therapy findings.[93–95] Because of the vast selection of cancer treatments with differing beneficial, toxicity, and cost profiles, ASCO formed a value framework to utilize for shared-decision making conversations with patients and clinicians for different treatment options.[94] There are two instruments, one for advanced disease and another for potentially curable disease (adjuvant therapy), with each incorporating the regimen's clinical benefit, toxicity, and effect on quality of life based on clinical trial results and cost.

Readers should look for authors to discuss previous findings regarding the topic of investigation and compare the study's results to literature that has been previously published. This practice allows for comparing results across multiple reports and conducting meta-analyses to achieve stronger confidence in findings pertaining to a certain topic.[69]

Readers should confirm that study conclusions stated in the article are truly supported by results and then decide if the results are clinically relevant. Once the findings seem clinically important and valid, the question can be asked of whether the findings are important in caring for a certain patient population. One question is whether the study participants and target population are similar enough to one's clinical patients. The second is whether applying the test, intervention, or other change in practice is feasible in a particular clinical setting.

Conclusion

There has been a large expansion in studies using big data—primarily large clinical or administrative datasets—over the past 15 years. These types of studies have the potential to help inform and change clinical practice when conducted and interpreted appropriately. We reviewed the advantages of big data studies and what areas of research and situations it may most successfully used for, including describing disease processes (including infrequent events) and treatments, evaluating diagnostic practices, and provide information regarding disparities that highlight gaps in delivering quality and equitable care. We also discussed the pitfalls of big data in otolaryngology and best practices when interpreting big data literature, emphasizing the fact that the pitfalls discussed can affect all research and are not unique to big data. The pitfalls include selection bias, observation bias, missing data, confounding, immortal time bias, and discerning statistical versus clinical significance. If clinicians do not think critically and consider pitfalls when reading and interpreting studies, applying big data findings to clinical practice could lead to worse patient outcomes. Some of the pitfalls may be mitigated by scrutinizing methods of papers including the flow diagrams of patient inclusion and exclusion criteria and strategy and remaining cognizant of the difference between statistical and clinical significance. Applying big data research to clinical practice requires following a purposeful intake strategy of literature, noting the objectives and reading accordingly, remaining cognizant of sources of biases while avoiding research nihilism, and applying the findings to clinical patients and practice.

References

1. Subbarayan RS, Koester L, Villwock MR, Villwock J. Proliferation and contributions of national database studies in otolaryngology literature published in the United States: 2005−2016. *Ann Otol Rhinol Laryngol*. 2018;127(9):643−648.
2. Childers CP, Maggard-Gibbons M. Same data, opposite results?: a call to improve surgical database research. *JAMA Surg*. 2021;156(3):219−220.
3. Kaper NM, Swart KMA, Grolman W, Van Der Heijden G. Quality of reporting and risk of bias in therapeutic otolaryngology publications. *J Laryngol Otol*. 2018;132(1):22−28.
4. Gettelfinger JD, Paulk PB, Schmalbach CE. Patient safety and quality improvement. *Otolaryngology-Head Neck Surg (Tokyo)*. 2021;165(1_suppl):P46−P54.
5. Densen P. Challenges and opportunities facing medical education. *Trans Am Clin Climatol Assoc*. 2011;122:48−58.
6. Schneeweiss S, Avorn J. A review of uses of health care utilization databases for epidemiologic research on therapeutics. *J Clin Epidemiol*. 2005;58(4):323−337.

7. Suissa S. Immortal time bias in pharmaco-epidemiology. *Am J Epidemiol*. 2008;167(4):492−499.
8. Fields AC, Lu P, Palenzuela DL, et al. Does retrieval bag use during laparoscopic appendectomy reduce postoperative infection? *Surgery*. 2019;165(5):953−957.
9. Turner SA, Jung HS, Scarborough JE. Utilization of a specimen retrieval bag during laparoscopic appendectomy for both uncomplicated and complicated appendicitis is not associated with a decrease in postoperative surgical site infection rates. *Surgery*. 2019;165(6):1199−1202.
10. Childers CP, Maggard-Gibbons M. Re: does retrieval bag use during laparoscopic appendectomy reduce postoperative infection? *Surgery*. 2019;166(1):127−128.
11. Jones EA, Shuman AG, Egleston BL, Liu JC. Common pitfalls of head and neck research using cancer registries. *Otolaryngol Head Neck Surg*. 2019;161(2):245−250.
12. Smith AM, Chaiet SR. Big data in facial plastic and reconstructive surgery: from large databases to registries. *Curr Opin Otolaryngol Head Neck Surg*. 2017;25(4):273−279.
13. Tang AB, Childers CP, Dworsky JQ, Maggard-Gibbons M. Surgeon work captured by the national surgical quality improvement program across specialties. *Surgery*. 2020;167(3):550−555.
14. Raval MV, Pawlik TM. Practical guide to surgical data sets: national surgical quality improvement program (NSQIP) and pediatric NSQIP. *JAMA Surg*. 2018;153(8):764−765.
15. Chung SY, Unsal AA, Kılıç S, Baredes S, Liu JK, Eloy JA. Pediatric sinonasal malignancies: a population-based analysis. *Int J Pediatr Otorhinolaryngol*. 2017;98:97−102.
16. Bilimoria KY, Liu Y, Paruch JL, et al. Development and evaluation of the universal ACS NSQIP surgical risk calculator: a decision aid and informed consent tool for patients and surgeons. *J Am Coll Surg*. 2013;217(5):833−842.
17. Burton BN, Jafari A, Asmerom B, Swisher MW, Gabriel RA, DeConde A. Inpatient mortality after endoscopic sinus surgery for invasive fungal rhinosinusitis. *Ann Otol Rhinol Laryngol*. 2019;128(4):300−308.
18. Simmonds JC, Vecchiotti M. Cholesteatoma as a complication of Langerhans Cell Histiocytosis of the temporal bone: a nationwide cross-sectional analysis. *Int J Pediatr Otorhinolaryngol*. 2017;100:66−70.
19. Hamdi OA, Jonas RH, Daniero JJ. Vocal Fold paralysis following COVID-19 vaccination: query of VAERS database. *J Voice*. 2022. https://doi.org/10.1016/j.jvoice.2022.01.016.
20. Shay AD, Zaniletti I, Davis KP, Bolin E, Richter GT. Characterizing pediatric bilateral Vocal fold dysfunction: analysis with the pediatric health information system database. *Laryngoscope*. 2022;133:1228−1233.
21. Reid L, Carroll W. Treacher collins syndrome in the United States: examining incidence and inpatient interventions. *Cleft Palate Craniofac J*. 2021;58(11):1438−1442.
22. McCoul ED, Weinreich HM, Mulder H, Man LX, Schulz K, Shin JJ. Health care utilization and prescribing patterns for adult eustachian tube dysfunction. *Otolaryngol Head Neck Surg*. 2019;160(6):1071−1080.
23. Alexander M, Ray MA, Hébert JR, et al. The national veteran sleep disorder study: descriptive epidemiology and secular trends, 2000−2010. *Sleep*. 2016;39(7):1399−1410.
24. Barnes JM, Graboyes EM, Adjei Boakye E, et al. The Affordable care act and suicide incidence among adults with cancer. *J Cancer Surviv*. 2022;17:449−459.

25. Smolinski NE, Antonelli PJ, Winterstein AG. Watchful waiting for acute otitis media. *Pediatrics*. 2022;150(1).

26. Jin MC, Qian ZJ, Cooperman SP, Alyono JC. Trends in use and timing of intratympanic corticosteroid injections for sudden sensorineural hearing loss. *Otolaryngol Head Neck Surg*. 2021;165(1):166−173.

27. Huang Z, Gordish-Dressman H, Preciado D, Reilly BK. Pediatric cochlear implantation: variation in income, race, payer, and charges across five states. *Laryngoscope*. 2018; 128(4):954−958.

28. Mullen MC, Yan F, Ford ME, Patel KG, Pecha PP. Racial and ethnic disparities in primary cleft lip and cleft palate repair. *Cleft Palate Craniofac J*. 2021;60:482−488.

29. Zhu VZ, Tuggle CT, Au AF. Promise and limitations of big data research in plastic surgery. *Ann Plast Surg*. 2016;76(4):453−458.

30. Kamarajah SK, Nathan H. Strengths and limitations of registries in surgical oncology research. *J Gastrointest Surg*. 2021;25(11):2989−2996.

31. Adams ME, Karaca-Mandic P, Marmor S. Use of neuroimaging for patients with dizziness who present to outpatient clinics vs emergency departments in the US. *JAMA Otolaryngol Head Neck Surg*. 2022;148(5):465−473.

32. Jang DW, Lee HJ, Chen PG, Cohen SM, Scales CD. Geographic variations in healthcare utilization and expenditure for chronic rhinosinusitis: a population-based approach. *Laryngoscope*. 2021;131(12):2641−2648.

33. Wang W, Krishnan E. Big data and clinicians: a review on the state of the science. *JMIR Med Inform*. 2014;2(1):e1.

34. Wick EH, Deutsch B, Kallogjeri D, Chi JJ, Branham GH. Effectiveness of prophylactic preoperative antibiotics in mandible fracture repair: a national database study. *Otolaryngol Head Neck Surg*. 2021;165(6):798−808.

35. Moroco AE, Saadi RA, Patel VA, Lehman EB, Gniady JP. 30-Day postoperative outcomes following transcervical Zenker's diverticulectomy in the elderly: analysis of the NSQIP database. *Otolaryngol Head Neck Surg*. 2021;165(1):129−136.

36. Youn GM, Shah JP, Wei EX, Kandathil C, Most SP. Revision rates of septoplasty in the United States. *Facial Plast Surg Aesthet Med*. 2022;25:153−158.

37. Ibrahim B, de Freitas Mendonca MI, Gombar S, Callahan A, Jung K, Capasso R. Association of systemic diseases with surgical treatment for obstructive sleep apnea compared with continuous positive Airway pressure. *JAMA Otolaryngol Head Neck Surg*. 2021; 147(4):329−335.

38. Kulaylat AS, Schaefer EW, Messaris E, Hollenbeak CS. Truven health analytics MarketScan databases for clinical research in colon and rectal surgery. *Clin Colon Rectal Surg*. 2019;32(1):54−60.

39. Institute NC. Surveillance, epidemiology, and end results program. 2020.

40. Sheils CR, Dahlke AR, Kreutzer L, Bilimoria KY, Yang AD. Evaluation of hospitals participating in the American College of surgeons national surgical quality improvement program. *Surgery*. 2016;160(5):1182−1188.

41. Mazul AL, Hartman CM, Mowery YM, et al. Risk and incidence of head and neck cancers in veterans living with HIV and matched HIV-negative veterans. *Cancer*. 2022; 128(18):3310−3318.

42. Bur AM, Villwock MR, Nallani R, et al. National database research in head and neck reconstructive surgery: a call for increased transparency and reproducibility. *Otolaryngol Head Neck Surg*. 2021;164(2):315−321.

43. Drinane JJ, Drinane J, Nair L, Patel A. Head and neck reconstruction: does surgical specialty affect complication rates? *J Reconstr Microsurg.* 2019;35(7):516−521.

44. Graboyes EM, Garrett-Mayer E, Ellis MA, et al. Effect of time to initiation of postoperative radiation therapy on survival in surgically managed head and neck cancer. *Cancer.* 2017;123(24):4841−4850.

45. Parsons HM, Henderson WG, Ziegenfuss JY, Davern M, Al-Refaie WB. Missing data and interpretation of cancer surgery outcomes at the American College of surgeons national surgical quality improvement program. *J Am Coll Surg.* 2011;213(3):379−391.

46. Deal JA, Gross AL, Sharrett AR, et al. Hearing impairment and missing cognitive test scores in a population-based study of older adults: the Atherosclerosis Risk in Communities neurocognitive study. *Alzheimers Dement.* 2021;17(10):1725−1734.

47. Piccillo EM, Adkins D, Elrakhawy M, Carr MM. Cricopharyngeal myotomy in national surgical quality improvement program (NSQIP): complications for otolaryngologists versus non-otolaryngologists. *Cureus.* 2021;13(10):e19021.

48. Quimby AE, Grose E, Reddy D, Webster R, Malic C, Vaccani JP. Predictors of surgical site infection in pediatric cochlear implantation. *Otolaryngol Head Neck Surg.* 2022:1945998221104933.

49. Garber D, Wandell GM, Gobillot TA, Merati A, Bhatt NK, Giliberto JP. Safety and predictors of 30-day adverse events of laryngeal framework surgery: an analysis of ACS-NSQIP data. *Laryngoscope.* 2022;132(7):1414−1420.

50. Schneider AL, Lavin JM. Publicly available databases in otolaryngology quality improvement. *Otolaryngol Clin North Am.* 2019;52(1):185−194.

51. Prasad KG, Nelson BG, Deig CR, Schneider AL, Moore MG. ACS NSQIP risk calculator: an accurate predictor of complications in major head and neck surgery? *Otolaryngol Head Neck Surg.* 2016;155(5):740−742.

52. Helman SN, Brant JA, Moubayed SP, Newman JG, Cannady SB, Chai RL. Predictors of length of stay, reoperation, and readmission following total laryngectomy. *Laryngoscope.* 2017;127(6):1339−1344.

53. Perry A, Kerezoudis P, Graffeo CS, et al. Little insights from big data: cerebrospinal fluid leak after skull base surgery and the limitations of database research. *World Neurosurg.* 2019;127:e561−e569.

54. Bollig CA, Morris B, Stubbs VC. Transoral robotic surgery with neck dissection versus nonsurgical treatment in stage I and II human papillomavirus-negative oropharyngeal cancer. *Head Neck.* 2022;44(7):1545−1553.

55. Randhawa A, Randhawa KS, Tseng CC, Fang CH, Baredes S, Eloy JA. Racial disparities in charges, length of stay, and complications following adult inpatient epistaxis treatment. *Am J Rhinol Allergy.* 2022;37:51−57.

56. Boffa DJ, Rosen JE, Mallin K, et al. Using the national cancer database for outcomes research: a review. *JAMA Oncol.* 2017;3(12):1722−1728.

57. Stitzenberg KB, Chang Y, Smith AB, Nielsen ME. Exploring the burden of inpatient readmissions after major cancer surgery. *J Clin Oncol.* 2015;33(5):455−464.

58. Freeman RK, Dilts JR, Ascioti AJ, Dake M, Mahidhara RS. A comparison of length of stay, readmission rate, and facility reimbursement after lobectomy of the lung. *Ann Thorac Surg.* 2013;96(5):1740−1745.

59. Stitzenberg KB, Chang Y, Smith AB, Meyers MO, Nielsen ME. Impact of location of readmission on outcomes after major cancer surgery. *Ann Surg Oncol.* 2017;24(2):319−329.

60. Weiss NS. The new world of data linkages in clinical epidemiology: are we being brave or foolhardy? *Epidemiology.* 2011;22(3):292−294.

61. Kim DH, Schneeweiss S. Measuring frailty using claims data for pharmacoepidemiologic studies of mortality in older adults: evidence and recommendations. *Pharmacoepidemiol Drug Saf.* 2014;23(9):891−901.

62. Brookhart MA, Stürmer T, Glynn RJ, Rassen J, Schneeweiss S. Confounding control in healthcare database research: challenges and potential approaches. *Med Care.* 2010;48(6 Suppl):S114−S120.

63. Cole KL, Babajanian E, Anderson R, et al. Association of baseline frailty status and age with postoperative complications after cochlear implantation: a national inpatient sample study. *Otol Neurotol.* 2022;43:1170−1175.

64. Zanation AM, Carrau RL, Snyderman CH, et al. Nasoseptal flap reconstruction of high flow intraoperative cerebral spinal fluid leaks during endoscopic skull base surgery. *Am J Rhinol Allergy.* 2009;23(5):518−521.

65. Mehta GU, Oldfield EH. Prevention of intraoperative cerebrospinal fluid leaks by lumbar cerebrospinal fluid drainage during surgery for pituitary macroadenomas. *J Neurosurg.* 2012;116(6):1299−1303.

66. Snyderman CH, Janecka IP, Sekhar LN, Sen CN, Eibling DE. Anterior cranial base reconstruction: role of galeal and pericranial flaps. *Laryngoscope.* 1990;100(6): 607−614.

67. Lucas DJ, Haider A, Haut E, et al. Assessing readmission after general, vascular, and thoracic surgery using ACS-NSQIP. *Ann Surg.* 2013;258(3):430−439.

68. Lucas DJ, Haut ER, Hechenbleikner EM, Wick EC, Pawlik TM. Avoiding immortal time bias in the American College of surgeons national surgical quality improvement program readmission measure. *JAMA Surg.* 2014;149(8):875−877.

69. Piccirillo JF. Improving the quality of the reporting of research results. *JAMA Otolaryngol Head Neck Surg.* 2016;142(10):937−939.

70. Kou YF, Wang C, Shah GB, Mitchell RB, Johnson RF. Tonsillectomy outcomes among children with mental health disorders in the United States. *Otolaryngol Head Neck Surg.* 2020;162(5):754−760.

71. Favre N, Patel VA, Carr MM. Complications in pediatric acute mastoiditis: HCUP KID analysis. *Otolaryngol Head Neck Surg.* 2021;165(5):722−730.

72. Karadaghy OA, Hong H, Scott-Wittenborn N, et al. Reporting of effect size and confidence Intervals in JAMA otolaryngology-head & neck surgery. *JAMA Otolaryngol Head Neck Surg.* 2017;143(11):1075−1080.

73. Piccirillo JF, Mager DE, Frisse ME, Brophy RH, Goggin A. Impact of first-line vs second-line antibiotics for the treatment of acute uncomplicated sinusitis. *JAMA.* 2001;286(15):1849−1856.

74. Nathan H, Pawlik TM. Limitations of claims and registry data in surgical oncology research. *Ann Surg Oncol.* 2008;15(2):415−423.

75. Schober P, Bossers SM, Schwarte LA. Statistical significance versus clinical importance of observed effect sizes: what do P values and confidence Intervals really represent? *Anesth Analg.* 2018;126(3):1068−1072.

76. Neely JG, Paniello RC, Nussenbaum B, Engel SH, Karni RJ, Fraley PL. Practical guides to efficient life-long learning. *Otolaryngol Head Neck Surg.* 2006;135(4):608−615.

77. Rudmik L, Xu Y, Alt JA, et al. Evaluating surgeon-specific performance for endoscopic sinus surgery. *JAMA Otolaryngol Head Neck Surg.* 2017;143(9):891−898.

78. Zumsteg ZS, Luu M, Yoshida EJ, et al. Combined high-intensity local treatment and systemic therapy in metastatic head and neck squamous cell carcinoma: an analysis of the National Cancer Data Base. *Cancer*. 2017;123(23):4583−4593.

79. Connell FA, Diehr P, Hart LG. The use of large data bases in health care studies. *Annu Rev Public Health*. 1987;8:51−74.

80. Ho AS, Kim S, Tighiouart M, et al. Metastatic lymph node burden and survival in oral cavity cancer. *J Clin Oncol*. 2017;35(31):3601−3609.

81. van Walraven C, Austin P. Administrative database research has unique characteristics that can risk biased results. *J Clin Epidemiol*. 2012;65(2):126−131.

82. Goel AN, Frangos MI, Raghavan G, et al. The impact of treatment package time on survival in surgically managed head and neck cancer in the United States. *Oral Oncol*. 2019; 88:39−48.

83. Graboyes EM, Kallogjeri D, Saeed MJ, Olsen MA, Nussenbaum B. 30-day hospital readmission following otolaryngology surgery: analysis of a state inpatient database. *Laryngoscope*. 2017;127(2):337−345.

84. Hoskin TL, Boughey JC, Day CN, Habermann EB. Lessons learned regarding missing clinical stage in the national cancer database. *Ann Surg Oncol*. 2019;26(3):739−745.

85. Kahlert J, Gribsholt SB, Gammelager H, Dekkers OM, Luta G. Control of confounding in the analysis phase - an overview for clinicians. *Clin Epidemiol*. 2017;9:195−204.

86. Yan F, Li H, de Almeida JR, et al. Microscopic extranodal extension in HPV-negative head and neck cancer and the role of adjuvant chemoradiation. *Otolaryngol Head Neck Surg*. 2021;165(4):536−549.

87. Peters LJ, O'Sullivan B, Giralt J, et al. Critical impact of radiotherapy protocol compliance and quality in the treatment of advanced head and neck cancer: results from TROG 02.02. *J Clin Oncol*. 2010;28(18):2996−3001.

88. Pignon JP, le Maître A, Maillard E, Bourhis J. Meta-analysis of chemotherapy in head and neck cancer (MACH-NC): an update on 93 randomised trials and 17,346 patients. *Radiother Oncol*. 2009;92(1):4−14.

89. Strojan P, Vermorken JB, Beitler JJ, et al. Cumulative cisplatin dose in concurrent chemoradiotherapy for head and neck cancer: a systematic review. *Head Neck*. 2016; 38(Suppl 1):E2151−E2158.

90. Ho AS, Luu M, Barrios L, et al. Prognostic impact of histologic grade for papillary thyroid carcinoma. *Ann Surg Oncol*. 2021;28(3):1731−1739.

91. Best CAE, Quimby AE, Johnson-Obaseki S. Alternative sources of cautery may improve post-operative hematoma rates but increase operative time in thyroid surgery. *Sci Rep*. 2021;11(1):22569.

92. Etchill EW, Giuliano KA, Boss EF, Rhee DS, Kunisaki SM. Association of operative approach with outcomes in neonates with esophageal atresia and tracheoesophageal fistula. *J Pediatr Surg*. 2021;56(12):2172−2179.

93. Dahlberg SE, Korn EL, Le-Rademacher J, Mandrekar SJ. Clinical versus statistical significance in studies of thoracic malignancies. *J Thorac Oncol*. 2020;15(9):1406−1408.

94. Schnipper LE, Davidson NE, Wollins DS, et al. Updating the American society of clinical oncology value framework: revisions and reflections in response to comments received. *J Clin Oncol*. 2016;34(24):2925−2934.

95. Cherny NI, Dafni U, Bogaerts J, et al. ESMO-magnitude of clinical benefit Scale version 1.1. *Ann Oncol*. 2017;28(10):2340−2366.

Current big data approaches to clinical questions in otolaryngology

5

Nicholas A. Rapoport, BS [1], **Andrew P. Michelson, MD** [2,3] and **Matthew A. Shew, MD** [4]

[1]*School of Medicine, Washington University in St. Louis, St. Louis, MO, United States;* [2]*Department of Pulmonary Critical Care, Washington University School of Medicine, St. Louis, MO, United States;* [3]*Institute for Informatics, Data Science & Biostatistics, Washington University School of Medicine, St. Louis, MO, United States;* [4]*Department of Otolaryngology-Head and Neck Surgery, Washington University School of Medicine in St. Louis, St. Louis, MO, United States*

Introduction

Over the last several decades, we have seen a cataclysmic shift in healthcare delivery from paper charts into an era of technological innovation, healthcare digitalization, and "Big data." In today's digital era, as more hospitals and clinics have implemented electronic health records (EHRs), the amount of data available to physicians, researchers, and scientists has skyrocketed and subsequently has transformed the way healthcare is delivered and how patient outcomes are assessed. The dissemination and implementation of EHRs across hospitals and clinics has led to the digitalization of granular information and is largely responsible for the rapid growth of big data in healthcare. EHRs, and other sources of data, such as medical insurance related databases, have led to huge repositories of raw data that is becoming increasingly complex both in volume and data dimensionality. These datasets are often stored in different formats, and are variably large and complex, rendering traditional analysis difficult.[1,2] It is estimated that there will be around one billion patient encounters documented per year in the United States alone.[3] The sheer amount of data from EHRs has the potential to revolutionize many aspects of healthcare if properly utilized, but properly utilizing the data from EHRs is complex and difficult. Modern healthcare informatics and data science approaches have emerged out of necessity, allowing clinicians, researchers, and administrators to transform this heterogenous and unorganized data into digestible and clinically relevant formats that can be readily understood, actionable, and outcome directed.[4]

The American Medical Informatics Association defines informatics as "the science of how to use data, information, and knowledge to improve human health and the delivery of health care services."[5] With the ever advancing field of clinical informatics alongside the expanding field of "Big data," we have seen a dramatic rise in

Big Data in Otolaryngology. https://doi.org/10.1016/B978-0-443-10520-3.00007-1

publications leveraging "Big Data" to help provide novel insights into otherwise elusive clinical and patient centric questions. Similarly, larger datasets have allowed clinicians and researchers to identify correlations and related data clusters to develop and implement innovative predictive models that can then translate directly to the bedside to aid and augment clinical decision making.[6] These innovative approaches have already influenced many fields of medicine. Data centric and artificial intelligence (AI) based approaches are helping physicians synthesize the data into an actionable form that can be integrated into clinical decisions in realtime.[4,7] These algorithms can also aid early detection and identification of diseases and likely could provide a benefit to all fields of medicine.[8]

Big data integration and utilization in otolaryngology is still in its infancy relative to other specialties in medicine. As we collectively move forward in understanding "Big Data" and its implications for clinical care, it is critical we understand where it has been applied already. It is equally important to recognize its relative strengths, weaknesses, and biases as we look to integrate "Big Data" into a clinical paradigm that assists in clinical decision making. This chapter will explore the general field of big data in otolaryngology, current big data sources used in otolaryngology, and how it has been and could further be leveraged to improve patient care.

Definitions in big data and how big data can be leveraged

Big data has become prevalent in many different fields, such as medicine, business, and law; however, there is a lack of a precise and rigid definition, as big data and its related concepts are constantly evolving. Big data has been defined as data that are generated in high volumes, high variety, and at a high velocity.[9,10] There are also recognized properties of big data, such as requiring computational infrastructure in order to process the data, and an inherent challenge on extracting meaningful information into digestible and actionable items.[11]

Definitions of big data are necessarily broad because big data is heterogenous in many aspects. Heterogeneity in big data can be seen in the variable depth and breadth of current big datasets. For example, EHRs often contain only a few elements per patient (depth) but become big data when there are millions of records (breadth).[12] The inverse is seen in new techniques utilized by "omics" fields such as genomics; next generation sequencing will produce millions of elements and becomes big data after only a few samples. Both are considered big data and require data science skillsets to extract knowledge from raw information.

Data science has been defined as "the set of fundamental principles that support and guide the principled extraction of information and knowledge from data."[8] Other important terms to define are data mining, AI, and machine learning. AI is an umbrella definition for multiple tasks (e.g., machine learning, natural language processing, etc.) that mimic human like intelligence, such as reasoning, problem solving, and knowledge representation, performed by machines at a speed and breadth that exceeds normal human capabilities.[13] Machine learning is a term that combines multiple forms of statistical models that allows computers to learn from labeled examples.[14] Data mining is the process of utilizing data science principles in combination with AI/machine learning to extract and derive meaningful information from the data.

It is important to recognize that the strength of these techniques is intrinsically linked to the quality of the data; this is currently one of the largest weaknesses of big data sourced from EHRs. Data documented in EHRs can be erroneous, miscoded, fragmented, and incomplete.[15,16] Studies have demonstrated that less than a quarter of all records are considered complete.[16] The data are also inherently susceptible to human error and biases from each individual who enters data on their respective patient encounters, and there is a lack of standardization on recording encounters and clinical data in the EHR.[17] These shortcomings are critical to always keep in the forethought not only when leveraging big data to help answer clinical questions and improve healthcare and precision medicine delivery but also as we collectively move forward and improve on current systems and shift toward personalized medicine.

Given the potential pitfalls of EHRs and, by extension, certain big datasets, it is critical to consider the proper way to collect and leverage big data in medicine. The massive amount of data and the collaborative nature of nationwide EHRs provide researchers with the ability to potentially generalize study results to a larger population, alleviating some bias seen in single institution studies that may only capture certain types of individuals. Big data also allows researchers to study rare pathologies that are otherwise unfeasible with single institution studies. Big data can discern extremely complex and subtle trends in outcomes, diseases, and treatment plans in a way that smaller databases simply cannot. This can lead researchers to elucidate potential avenues to improving patient care of specific populations that cannot be adequately studied without these databases or larger national datasets. For example, genomics has allowed patients with BRCA1 genotypes to be identified early and receive appropriate preventative and interventive care in a timely manner.[18]

Alongside big data, there has been an exponential rise in innovative approaches like AI and machine learning within healthcare. AI models require large quantities of data to be leveraged to become tuned enough for widespread adoption. Big data can provide this "training" and has been the stepping stone for these novel approaches. In return, AI has allowed us to enhance our modeling techniques, and newer AI innovations like deep neural networks can be applied to sources of data that inherently encode rich information (e.g., CT scans, MRI, electrophysiologic data, etc.). Certain fields, like critical care and oncology, are trailblazers within big data and improving clinical care models. For example, intensivists have significantly improved upon models predicting readmission to the intensive care unit by leveraging big data and machine learning.[19] While otolaryngology is starting to integrate big data to help answer evasive clinical questions and improve precision medicine delivery, the field is certainly naïve and in its early stages.

Most big data approaches to otolaryngology clinical questions are limited to different administrative and clinical registry datasets. These larger and national data sources provide many unique advantages given their size, use of EHR or claims data, and national scale. However, these datasets have their inherent biases and the data collected are not always otolaryngology centric. Other approaches that continue to gain traction within big data and otolaryngology include the use of EHR and large volumes of clinical data to improve precision medicine and predictive modeling. Another promising approach includes leveraging diverse and richer data sources such as imaging, genomic data, healthcare wearables, and electrophysiologic data.

As we progress and move forward with adopting clinical informatics into otolaryngology, it is critical we not only learn from what has been done and how it can improve patient care; it is essential we also work collectively to improve the quality of patient care through aggregation, harmonization, and analysis of big data with the goal of extracting actionable items that can further drive precision medicine.

Current databases and utilization in otolaryngology

Databases can largely be divided into two main subgroups: administrative/claims and clinical registries. Administrative datasets are compiled from codified information submitted for billing purposes. The EHR provides data via clinical providers or trained coders converting clinical information into numerical codes for diagnoses, procedures, and complications, typically using Internal Classification of Disease (ICD) or Current Procedural Terminology (CPT) codes. This information is then submitted to insurance companies for reimbursement. Administrative databases often use ICD and CPT based codes as the main source or clinical anchor to help pull related data. The large advantage is uniform definitions for either diagnosis codes or procedures input by clinical experts. Conversely, their limitations also reside in the fact that it is defined by clinical providers, their respective biases, and inherently retrospective nature.

Clinical registries, on the other hand, are built by clinically trained professionals collecting and entering data into the chart and are created and maintained for research purposes or quality improvement initiatives. Due to this, clinical registries have more detailed clinical information, and allow for a more specific focus in clinical areas than administrative databases. Clinical registries are by nature prospective and often have a significant forethought prior to implementation.

There is a plethora of both groups of databases; the purpose of this chapter is not to provide an exhaustive list of current databases, but to show how these databases are currently utilized to help answer clinical questions in otolaryngology. The remainder of this section will detail the advantages and disadvantages of administrative and clinical databases and give examples of recent research in otolaryngology and its subspecialties.

Administrative databases in otolaryngology

Since administrative databases are born from billing insurances, practically every patient encounter is captured by these databases, and the sheer amount of data lends a strong statistical advantage to them. Over the last decade, there has been a rapid rise in epidemiologic studies leveraging these databases. Administrative databases are also built from preexisting infrastructure, where a plethora of data can be pulled in a retrospective nature without additional cost to procure or maintain. One of the largest limitations with administrative databases is that ICD and CPT coding is directly connected to hospital and physician reimbursement, as well as other outcome metrics not directly related to patient care (e.g., hospital U.S News and Report rankings). Despite attempts to create more uniform criteria for billing, there remains heterogeneity in how physicians document patient encounters and how clinical information is coded for billing purposes. Unfortunately, this can lead to distortion of how the disease under investigation appears in administrative data. An illustration of how administrative databases are constructed is presented in Fig. 5.1.

Studies have shown mixed results in how accurate medical records are in relation to these codes; administrative datasets are often incomplete and inaccurate when verified with manual chart review. While some may accurately capture broad categories of disease, they often suffer from inaccuracy when trying to hone in on specific types of pathologies and therefore do not represent the true disease under investigation.[20–22] ICD codes are often reported to insurance companies as primary and secondary diagnoses, and attempts by physicians to accurately capture the severity of disease can lead to researchers having difficulty elucidating simple temporal trends.[23] For example, when a primary diagnosis of pneumonia is replaced with a primary diagnosis of sepsis and a secondary diagnosis of pneumonia, it can lead to drastic changes in overall pneumonia trends when aggregated across millions of encounters.[23] This is a significant challenge, given primary coding for sepsis is more severe and associated with higher reimbursement than pneumonia. Similarly for otolaryngology, when a primary diagnosis of acute otitis media is replaced with otomastoiditis complicated by meningitis for billing purposes, similar inaccuracies are captured. Additionally, many procedures are severely underreported due to a lack of financial incentive.[24] Conversely, procedures that are highly profitable will almost always be captured accurately and may appear to be overreported when compared to less profitable procedures.[25]

There are also limits to generalizability of administrative databases since the data source is a nonrandom sample, and patient populations are inevitably fragmented based on both clinical and socioeconomic demographics. For example, geographic and demographic profiles in private insurance databases will differ from the Centers for Medicare and Medicaid services (CMS) databases. The socioeconomic disparities from CMS, particularly Medicaid, will differ drastically from those that are privately insured. Furthermore, different insurance providers will have different eligibility criteria or rates of denial for various diagnoses or procedures. For example, cochlear implant candidacy and single sided deafness vary drastically, not only from various private insurance providers but also on a CMS level and Medicaid level from state to state. Private insurance databases may also be limited geographically, and patients with small health plans are often underrepresented. Importantly, data become unavailable after a change in health plan and limit the follow up data. This frequently occurs in the US due to geographic or employment

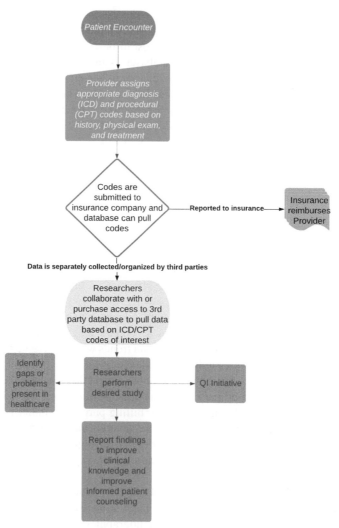

FIGURE 5.1

Illustration of how administrative datasets are built and used. *Abbreviations: CPT,* common procedural terminology; *ICD,* international classification of diseases; *QI,* quality improvement.

changes and other unavoidable circumstances. Finally, one of the largest barriers with administrative databases is prohibitive costs for researchers; for example, researchers desiring to utilize the private claims database MarketScan will pay upwards of $30,000 for access.

The general advantages and disadvantages of administrative databases are summarized in Table 5.1.

Table 5.1 Advantages and disadvantages of administrative databases.

Advantages	Disadvantages
Large amount of claims and related data	Can be biased due to heterogenous coding practices (under/overreporting of various procedures/complications)
No cost to build on the part of researcher; database will always exist due to requirements for reimbursement	Databases usually require paid access
Hypothesis generating by evaluating national trends or associations	May have less granular data (labs, comorbidities, outcomes [facial nerve, audiometric changes, etc.])
Generalizability based on geographic area captured and sample size	Demographic and socioeconomic bias may be present
Ability to study rare pathologies	Lack of follow up or outcome data

There are several publicly available administrative databases. The National Inpatient Sample (NIS) is the largest all payer inpatient care database and it captures between five and eight million patients per year, which represents approximately 20% of all US hospitalizations.[26] Similarly, the Kids' Inpatient Database (KID) is a publicly available, pediatric specific all payer database that captures over three million inpatient stays for patients under 21 years of age.[27] One of the most widely known administrative databases comes from CMS, which captures approximately 98% of adults 65 years and older enrolled in Medicare (over 65 million patients).[28] Finally, given the almost never ending amount of data, there are increasing numbers of commercially available services such as PearlDiver, IBM MarketScan, and IQVA.[29-31]

KID database and associated studies

The KID database offers unique insight as one of the largest pediatric databases. The data include several metrics specific to pediatric research: age in months for children under 10 years of age, complicated/uncomplicated birth, and hospital level classification (pediatric hospital, specialty pediatric hospital, not a pediatric hospital, or children's unit in a general hospital).[27] The KID has been used to study many otolaryngology specific issues, particularly in laryngology and airway surgery, and the huge amount of data allows for the analysis of rare pathologies otherwise unavailable in single institution studies. For example, it has allowed researchers to critically study cleft lip/palate repair in patients with hypopituitarism and showed these patients have a longer hospital course with increased complications than patients without hypopituitarism.[32] Pediatric thyroidectomies are rare compared to adults; however, a study utilizing the KID aggregated over 2700 thyroidectomy patients and demonstrated postoperative hypocalcemia occurred in up to 20% of pediatric patients, suggesting similar rates to their adult counterparts and supporting the need for established postoperative calcium supplementation.[33] Another study analyzed over 5300 tracheostomies in pediatric patients and found complications were elevated in younger children.[34] Rhinologists have utilized the KID to describe predisposing factors to invasive fungal sinusitis, common and rare complications of otitis media, how the rise of preoperative embolization of nasopharyngeal angiofibromas has positively affected outcomes, and demonstrate that chronic rhinosinusitis and cystic fibrosis are two of the most common comorbidities associated with morbidity or mortality following sinus surgery.[35–38].

The aforementioned studies highlight the ability of the KID, and other administrative databases, to study rare pathologies and rare outcomes in the field of otolaryngology. Searching PubMed for "kids inpatient database otolaryngology" leads to 93 results; these are selected examples to show how otolaryngologists have utilized the KID to improve patient care and gain insight on current issues that are more difficult to study using other databases or methods.

MarketScan and associated studies

MarketScan is a set of databases that are compiled and maintained by Truven Health Analytics. This data repository was launched as a quality improvement initiative in 1995 to improve oversight on healthcare cost effectiveness and maintain greater accountability.[29] A benefit of MarketScan is that it provides detailed data on prescription drug use and allows for quantification of healthcare costs; something that is notoriously difficult to study. Otologists have identified important factors associated with opioid misuse following tympanoplasty or mastoidectomy, while head and neck cancer surgeons found nearly 20% of patients develop chronic opioid use after surgery for laryngeal cancer.[39,40] Head and neck cancer surgeons have also shown economic burdens persist for at least 5 years after diagnosis and may disproportionately affect women.[41]

MarketScan has also been used to analyze trends in adoption of clinical care guidelines. For example, researchers demonstrated overall low rates of compliance for otitis media management recommendations on periods of watchful waiting.[42] Similarly, researchers have shown low adherence to oropharyngeal cancer guidelines for pretreatment imaging, thyroid function testing, and multidisciplinary consultation.[43] Another study used ICD codes and associated pharmaceutical prescription information to show poor adherence to Bell's palsy guidelines and treatment recommendations.[44] Finally, one study evaluated over 51,000 patients with chronic rhinosinusitis and showed wide variation in nonotolaryngology providers' management, and also illuminated how delayed referral to otolaryngology was strongly associated with increased healthcare costs.[45] This type of evidence provides substantiative grounds to advocate for earlier referral to improve healthcare cost utilization.

Databases built from claims data allow researchers to identify important opportunities for quality improvement measures. The examples of opioid pharmacotherapy, financial burden of cancer survivorship, and adoption of guidelines are just several examples identified here.

Clinical registries in otolaryngology

Clinical registries are created primarily for research specific purposes or quality improvement projects. By nature, these registries require more detailed clinical information to be recorded than administrative databases and are often intended to evaluate and improve outcomes for a population defined by a specific disease or exposure. Data are gathered prospectively in clinical registries by clinically trained reviewers, who abstract data from the medical record for patients included in the registry. These reviewers are trained in proper identification and coding of patient diagnoses, procedures, and outcomes, which leads to a higher fidelity information with fewer missed details. Researchers can therefore produce studies with more granular data than is available from administrative databases. Many subspecialties have several registries dedicated to patients of that subspecialty or with a particular pathology.[46] Clinical registries have several advantages for subspecialties, like otolaryngology, because outcome metrics and/or data can be gathered that are not standard of care and are not captured by larger administrative databases. An illustration of how clinical registries are created is presented in Fig. 5.2.

Since clinical registries almost always rely on manual data curation, clinical registries require intensive resources to establish and maintain. Clinical registries also vary in their breadth and depth; the National Surgical Quality Improvement Program (NSQIP) is one of the largest registries to date, and includes data from more than 600 hospitals across 49 states and nine countries.[47] Smaller registries that are built for particular pathologies, such as the American Burn Association Registry, or for a particular region, such as the Michigan Surgical Quality Collaborative, which may be less generalizable to the general population.[48]

The general advantages and disadvantages to clinical registries are presented in Table 5.2.

National surgical quality improvement program

One of the most prominent and published clinical registries is the NSQIP. The NSQIP was created in response to a federal mandate to improve quality assurance at Veteran Affairs (VA) hospitals by comparing outcomes to other surrounding community hospitals.[47] Due to its success, the NSQIP registry has now been implemented in more than 600 hospitals. These data are now used for studies for every surgical subspecialty, including otolaryngology. The NSQIP provides several insights for surgery related specialties because of its ability to not only track traditional clinical outcome data but also capture granular information on surgery (e.g., operative time, trainee involvement, 30 day complication rate, superficial versus deep infection, etc.) and also captures important outcome metrics (e.g., 30 day readmission rate, 30 day postoperative mortality, hospital length of stay, etc.). For example, one study was able to demonstrate that while resident participation did slightly increase operative time for both tympanoplasty, tympanomastoidectomy, thyroidectomy, and parathyroidectomy, there was no difference in complication rates.[49−51]

The NSQIP has found widespread application in otolaryngology. These data have been used by researchers to improve knowledge on facial reconstruction;

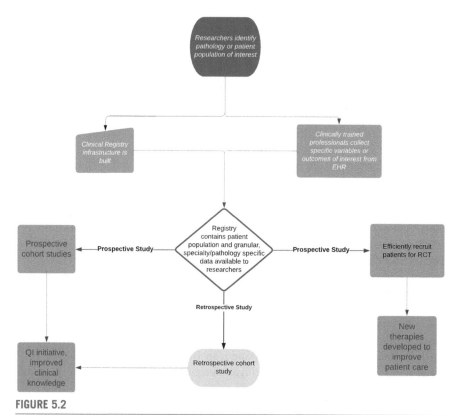

FIGURE 5.2

Illustration of how clinical registries are built and used. *Abbreviations*: *EHR*, electronic health record; *QI*, quality improvement; *RCT*, randomized controlled trial.

Table 5.2 Advantages and disadvantages of clinical registries.

Advantages	Disadvantages
Created explicitly for research/quality improvement	Resource intensive to establish infrastructure and maintain
Data gathered by professionals trained on particular disease states	Slower data collection with fewer patients
Can be created to serve a particular population or pathology	May be more difficult to generalize
Usually designed to be prospective	May have missing or incomplete data due to incomplete EHR documentation
Can put systems in place to assure quality data (e.g., NSQIP randomly audits sites to mitigate poor data)	Usually lack a control group for comparisons to a more general population
Can efficiently recruit patients for randomized controlled trials (RCTs)	

studies have elucidated predictive factors of paramedian forehead flap failure, demonstrated lower rates of short term complications in free flaps compared to pedicled flaps, and showed that patients with metabolic syndrome are at increased risk of sepsis and septic shock after head and neck reconstruction.[52−54] Rhinologists leveraged this source of big data to demonstrate the overall safety of endoscopic drainage of sinusitis related orbital complications, identify risk factors for admission following outpatient sinus surgery, and show exposure to cigarette smoke puts patients at a 4.5× increased risk for surgical site infections.[55−57] Neurotologists have studied common complications following schwannoma resection and also demonstrated that pediatric patients <3 years are at increased risk of readmission following otologic procedures.[58,59] Finally, otologists have demonstrated obesity has no impact on operative time, and therapeutic mastoidectomy in a chronic ear does not increase complication rates.[60,61] Collectively, the NSQIP has allowed otolaryngologists to study various surgery related complications and readmissions with huge sample sizes, allowing improved informed surgical decision making and improved patient counseling.

Historically controversial practices, such as septoplasty in younger pediatric patients, have been analyzed by leveraging the NSQIP and septoplasty was found to be safe and done more commonly in recent years.[62] Laryngomalacia procedures historically have had debates on risk factors for poor outcomes, but pediatric otolaryngologists addressed contradictory evidence by aggregating 1092 patients and elucidated that prematurity and pulmonary disease were the two most important factors associated with increased risk of postoperative complications and 30 day readmission.[63]

The NSQIP database can help to elucidate trends, risk factors, outcomes, and complications that would otherwise be missed by smaller scale studies and can inform clinicians about their practice. Searching PubMed for "NSQIP otolaryngology" produces 197 results. The selected examples offer only a few of the ways otolaryngologists have utilized this database. Many researchers have raised concerns that these large databases are being "abused" or inappropriately utilized. Given the large number of studies utilizing the NSQIP within Otolaryngology, it is critical providers analyze each study taking into consideration the strengths and weaknesses of the NSQIP, and how it is being applied to ensure conclusions are clinically relevant to patient care.

Reg ENT

The clinical registry Reg ENT is the first otolaryngology specific registry and was created by the American Academy of Otolaryngology Head and Neck Surgery/ Foundation (AAO HNSF) to focus on improving safety and care of otolaryngology patients.[64] This was created since most larger registries fail to capture otolaryngology specific outcomes. Reg ENT is relatively new and was first opened to general membership in July 2016. A great example of how Reg ENT can help address otolaryngology specific issues is a recent implementation of quality improvement initiatives in the treatment and diagnosis of age related hearing loss (ARHL).[65] Authors implemented four quality measures to help standardize protocols for both the diagnosis and treatment of AHRL; these include implementing hearing loss screening, audiometric referral and evaluation, guidelines on appropriate imaging work up, and shared risk decision making when pursuing treatment options. This represents a detailed example of how Reg ENT can be utilized for dissemination and implementation of novel protocols, and how Reg ENT can be implemented to help track quality improvement initiatives over a long term period. Another example is the collaboration between the American Academy of Neurology and the AAO HNSF to capture measures specific to benign paroxysmal positional vertigo.[66] While there are not currently many studies leveraging Reg ENT to help address critical questions in otolaryngology, Reg ENT is an exciting initiative and opportunity for otolaryngology researchers to be involved at the ground level, to help build the infrastructure toward big data specific to otolaryngology.

Growing innovative big data approaches in otolaryngology

There is an exciting amount of innovation harnessing big data and leveraging AI within otolaryngology. However, otolaryngology is still in its infancy regarding these novel approaches compared to other medical specialties. One of the largest rate limiting steps inhibiting its growth is the lack of otolaryngology centric datasets. This includes insufficient clinical and EHR data as well as a paucity of richer and more complex data such as imaging and genomics. Reg ENT is taking the necessary steps toward collaboration but will need time. Meanwhile, we have seen a rise in multiinstitutional collaborations seeking to build and improve otolaryngology centric big data and apply innovative AI computational techniques. For example, large collaboration in building audiometric and cochlear implant registry has allowed investigators to improve imputation models and boost sample sizes up to 5743 audiograms and 4739 cochlear implant recipients.[67,68] Similarly, multiinstitutional collaboration has allowed researchers to pool 2489 CI recipients to compare and contrast different prediction models.[69] Another study leveraged large audiometric datasets to build a quicker online audiogram using a machine learning Bayesian model with similar accuracy to a conventional audiogram.[70] Within head and neck, researchers pooled over 634 patients with oral cavity squamous cell carcinoma to apply machine learning based models to better predict occult nodal metastasis in N0 disease.[71] While these larger datasets and approaches offer significant promise, these are still relatively smaller datasets for AI based approach and there remains significant room for future opportunity.

Imaging data has offered novel avenues of improving personalized medicine by leveraging deep neural networks. Examples include using CT scans to help diagnose osteometal complex disease in patients with possible sinusitis, utilizing MRI to assess cortical predictors of language outcomes in pediatric cochlear implant recipients, and whether machine learning can help improve diagnosis of benign versus cancerous laryngeal lesions on laryngoscopy.[72−74] However, these exciting techniques are still in their preliminary phases. In the listed examples, external validation was done on smaller datasets and imaging data was not standardized, introducing several limitations and potential biases. A recent meta analysis pulled over 16 studies evaluating ear pathologies and shows significant promise with accuracies ranging from 76% to 98% accuracy; however, its generalizability is significantly limited by lack of standardized image protocols.[75]

Healthcare wearable devices are also providing unique opportunities within otolaryngology to use large, personalized datasets to revolutionize how we treat speech and hearing disorders. Deep neural networks may enable researchers to develop innovative hearing aids that transform components of sound into their "normal" neural representation, instead of simply amplifying and compressing sound, like current hearing aids do.[76] Conversely, it is possible to translate cortical neural information into speech; current brain—computer interfaces allow for slow, letter by letter selection, but a prototype of a neuroprosthesis utilizing AI has allowed a patient to communicate with triple the amount of words per minute and higher accuracy.[77] Additionally, researchers have used information gathered through hearing aids to better understand personal, behavioral, environmental, and other factors to better optimize fitting and end user utilization.[78] AI has improved cochlear implantation by using individual patient maps and utilization data to improve both personalized fitting strategies and implant outcomes.[79] Healthcare wearables and their massive amounts of personalized data offer a novel approach to otolaryngology and communication specific clinical dilemmas. While promising and exciting, significant work is still required to better capture and harmonize this potential data into actionable items.

Finally, with recent advancements in genomic sequencing and profiling, there is a significant push toward precision medicine utilizing individual patients' genome or biomarkers to deliver individualized care. Within hearing healthcare research, investigators have been leveraging tools like next generation sequencing panels to better understand individual patient pathologies.[80] Similarly, there is increased interest in using microRNAs and mass spectrometry to elucidate individual proteomic profiles within perilymph or blood in patients with varying hearing related diseases.[81—83] However, there remains a significant amount of work to better deliver gene therapies and other therapeutic measures, and to tailor genomic specific information to individual personalized treatment algorithms. Within head and neck cancer, the genomic landscape and key epigenetic markers are being rapidly uncovered at an unprecedent rate, allowing teams to better personalize cancer therapeutics.[84] Like many fields of oncology, big data within head and neck cancer genomes will undoubtedly further unfold into a "molecular tumor board" and allow providers to tailor individual recommendations and treatment plans.[85] A summary of selected innovations utilizing big data approaches is presented in Table 5.3.

The future of big data in otolaryngology

While there are multiple sources of big data that can help researchers address critical questions in otolaryngology, it is also evident there are several advantages and disadvantages. The future is bright; advanced technologies and computational power

Table 5.3 Summary of selected innovative big data approaches in otolaryngology.

Specialty	Application	Next steps
Otology/ Neurotology	• Assess cortical predictors of language outcomes in pediatric CI recipients using deep learning on MRI images	• Increase sample sizes. • Improve generalizability through external and prospective validation. • Evaluate other functional imaging modalities. • Assess complimentary role with other predictors of CI performance.
Laryngology, Head and Neck	• Machine Learning to predict occult metastasis • Deep learning to improve laryngeal lesion diagnosis (benign versus cancerous)	• Improve generalizability through external and prospective validation. • Standardize image protocols. • Assess attitudes, beliefs, and perceptions of how providers can use to complement clinical decision making. • Integrate genomic and/or pathologic data into models.
Otology/ Neurotology	• Develop hearing aids that transmit sound into neural representation • Develop neuroprosthesis that translate cortical activity into speech	• Increase scale of neural activity recordings to accurately characterize individuals. • Expand utilization of these innovative neuroprosthesis to enable larger sample sizes.
Head and Neck	• Utilize genomic sequencing and other biomarkers to deliver personalized treatment (i.e., personalized genomic tumor board)	• Build and improve collaborations that compliment clinical and genomic data across institutions. • Build multiinstitutional and longitudinal data repositories. • Increase the dissemination and implementation of genomic precision medicine delivery in head and neck cancer care.
Rhinology	Deep learning to improve clinically relevant CT diagnosis	• Increase sample sizes. • Improve generalizability through external and prospective validation. • Standardize image protocols.

Otology/ Neurotology	• Healthcare wearables and personalization
	  • Cochlear implant personalized mapping
	  • Hearing aid personalization
		• Improve healthcare wearable, clinical, data acquisition repositories.
		• Improve harmonization with longitudinal outcomes.

have allowed providers to better collect, analyze, and harmonize big data from clinical databases, EHRs, images, and genomic data. As we move forward, it is critical we analyze what has been done and what we can do moving forward to ensure we optimize our big data approaches. One of the most pressing issues facing these big data repositories is the quality of the data and collaboration across institutions. There is a profound lack of standardization in how clinical data are reported, stored, cleaned, curated, and transmitted, which diminishes the impact big data can currently have on medical and surgical practices. At the NIH level, new policies are now in place to better improve data repositories and sharing of scientific data.[86] However, big data organization is a significant challenge, and current NIH policies have been more reactive instead of proactive. Few funding mechanisms exist or incentivize big data organization and curation, and most of the innovation has been within the private sector. Ophthalmology has seen some of the largest private growth, where multiple companies have secured a massive series of funding as image based storage repositories and leveraging AI deep neural network based technologies into point of care screening tools.[87−89] The Observational Medical Outcomes Partnership (OMOP) is a public−private partnership that has recognized and attempted to mitigate this pitfall by implementing a common data model (CDM) to provide a single observational data schema that provides a comprehensive blueprint for data harmonization and sharing.[90] In essence, the CDM seeks to transform heterogenous data from EHRs into a common format by using standardized vocabulary and terminologies. These common formats will then enable systematic analysis. Adoption of a CDM will also allow specialty specific registries to cater to variables of unique interest to their specialty. An illustration of the CDM is presented in Fig. 5.3.

Another important consideration of big data is widespread adoption of the registries. Efficient integration of these registries into clinical workflow is critical in this regard. An editorial written by several of the creators of Reg ENT pointed out the necessity of actionable, timely, and accessible data specific to otolaryngological care, and noted Reg ENT is still lacking in these areas.[91] Currently, Reg ENT is a promising scaffold for quality improvement in otolaryngology, and strong participation is critical to its flourishment. A 2020 study found over 1600 providers were enrolled in Reg ENT, and the registry encompassed nearly 6.5 million unique patients and over 24 million patient encounters.[92] This is a strong start for powerful cohort studies, clinical trials, and prospective investigations, but the authors also identified a lack of diversity within the registry, which was partially due to a temporary inability to integrate local EHR vendor data into Reg ENT. As these roadblocks to adoption are identified and addressed, and as more providers contribute and participate to the body of data, Reg ENT will offer a tantalizingly powerful tool to the field of otolaryngology and precision medicine.

There is increasing evidence that these big data databases have the potential to revolutionize healthcare, provide insights into specific patient populations or pathologies, and ultimately improve personalized medicine. It is imperative that these tools

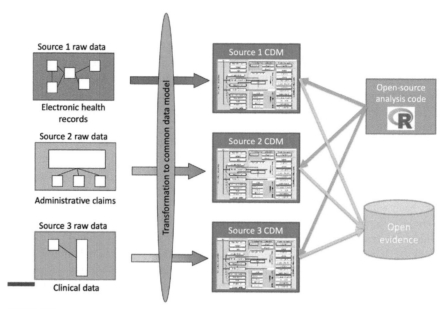

FIGURE 5.3

Illustration of the OMOP CDM (https://www.ohdsi.org/wp-content/uploads/2021/12/EMA-OHDSI-5-yr-review-Ryan-30nov2021.pdf).

are used accurately and appropriately. With millions of datapoints included in analysis, it is easy for conclusions to be misinterpreted due to poor data quality, poor analysis, or an inappropriately broad hypothesis. It is critical to mitigate these possibilities by ensuring accessible and accurate data that is widely available and actionable to physicians and researchers. In today's technological age, physicians must both utilize and contribute to these resources to provide quality care and improvements to patients' lives.

References

1. Ristevski B, Chen M. Big data analytics in medicine and healthcare. *J Integr Bioinform*. 2018;15(3):20170030. https://doi.org/10.1515/jib-2017-0030. Published 2018 May 10.
2. Kankanhalli A, Hahn J, Tan S, Gao G. Big data and analytics in healthcare: introduction to the special section. *Inf Syst Front*. 2016;18(2):233−235. https://doi.org/10.1007/s10796-016-9641-2.
3. Hripcsak G, Albers DJ. Next-generation phenotyping of electronic health records. *J Am Med Inf Assoc*. 2013;20(1):117−121. https://doi.org/10.1136/amiajnl-2012-001145.
4. Sanchez-Pinto LN, Luo Y, Churpek MM. Big data and data science in critical care. *Chest*. 2018;154(5):1239−1248. https://doi.org/10.1016/j.chest.2018.04.037.
5. https://amia.org/about-amia/why-informatics/informatics-research-and-practice.

6. Viceconti M, Hunter P, Hose R. Big data, big knowledge: big data for personalized healthcare. *IEEE J Biomed Health Inform*. 2015;19(4):1209–1215. https://doi.org/10.1109/JBHI.2015.2406883.

7. Schneider AL, Lavin JM. Publicly available databases in otolaryngology quality improvement. *Otolaryngol Clin North Am*. 2019;52(1):185–194. https://doi.org/10.1016/j.otc.2018.08.004.

8. Subrahmanya SVG, Shetty DK, Patil V, et al. The role of data science in healthcare advancements: applications, benefits, and future prospects. *Ir J Med Sci*. 2022;191(4):1473–1483. https://doi.org/10.1007/s11845-021-02730-z.

9. Provost F, Fawcett T. Data science and its relationship to big data and data-driven decision making. *Big Data*. 2013;1(1):51–59. https://doi.org/10.1089/big.2013.1508.

10. Bates DW, Saria S, Ohno-Machado L, Shah A, Escobar G. Big data in health care: using analytics to identify and manage high-risk and high-cost patients. *Health Aff*. 2014;33(7):1123–1131. https://doi.org/10.1377/hlthaff.2014.0041.

11. Baro E, Degoul S, Beuscart R, Chazard E. Toward a literature-driven definition of big data in healthcare. *BioMed Res Int*. 2015;2015:639021. https://doi.org/10.1155/2015/639021.

12. Obermeyer Z, Lee TH. Lost in thought - the limits of the human mind and the future of medicine. *N Engl J Med*. 2017;377(13):1209–1211. https://doi.org/10.1056/NEJMp1705348.

13. Stead WW. Clinical implications and challenges of artificial intelligence and deep learning. *JAMA*. 2018;320(11):1107–1108. https://doi.org/10.1001/jama.2018.11029.

14. Deo RC. Machine learning in medicine. *Circulation*. 2015;132(20):1920–1930. https://doi.org/10.1161/CIRCULATIONAHA.115.001593.

15. Hoffman S, Podgurski A. Big bad data: law, public health, and biomedical databases. *J Law Med Ethics*. 2013;41(Suppl 1):56–60. https://doi.org/10.1111/jlme.12040.

16. Weiskopf NG, Hripcsak G, Swaminathan S, Weng C. Defining and measuring completeness of electronic health records for secondary use. *J Biomed Inf*. 2013;46(5):830–836. https://doi.org/10.1016/j.jbi.2013.06.010.

17. Ross MK, Wei W, Ohno-Machado L. "Big data" and the electronic health record. *Yearb Med Inform*. 2014;9(1):97–104. https://doi.org/10.15265/IY-2014-0003. Published 2014 Aug 15.

18. Maddox TM, Rumsfeld JS, Payne PRO. Questions for artificial intelligence in health care. *JAMA*. 2019;321(1):31–32. https://doi.org/10.1001/jama.2018.18932.

19. Rojas JC, Carey KA, Edelson DP, Venable LR, Howell MD, Churpek MM. Predicting intensive care unit readmission with machine learning using electronic health record data. *Ann Am Thorac Soc*. 2018;15(7):846–853. https://doi.org/10.1513/AnnalsATS.201710-787OC.

20. Semins MJ, Trock BJ, Matlaga BR. Validity of administrative coding in identifying patients with upper urinary tract calculi. *J Urol*. 2010;184(1):190–192. https://doi.org/10.1016/j.juro.2010.03.011.

21. Woodworth GF, Baird CJ, Garces-Ambrossi G, Tonascia J, Tamargo RJ. Inaccuracy of the administrative database: comparative analysis of two databases for the diagnosis and treatment of intracranial aneurysms. *Neurosurgery*. 2009;65(2):251–257. https://doi.org/10.1227/01.NEU.0000347003.35690.7A.

22. Khwaja HA, Syed H, Cranston DW. Coding errors: a comparative analysis of hospital and prospectively collected departmental data. *BJU Int*. 2002;89(3):178–180. https://doi.org/10.1046/j.1464-4096.2001.01428.x.

23. Lindenauer PK, Lagu T, Shieh M, Pekow PS, Rothberg MB. Association of diagnostic coding with trends in hospitalizations and mortality of patients with pneumonia, 2003–2009. *JAMA*. 2012;307(13):1405–1413. https://doi.org/10.1001/jama.2012.384.

24. Haut ER, Pronovost PJ, Schneider EB. Limitations of administrative databases. *JAMA*. 2012;307(24):2589–2590. https://doi.org/10.1001/jama.2012.6626.

25. Sarrazin MS, Rosenthal GE. Finding pure and simple truths with administrative data. *JAMA*. 2012;307(13):1433–1435. https://doi.org/10.1001/jama.2012.404.

26. Agency for Healthcare Research Quality (AHRQ). *Agency for Healthcare Research Quality (ARHQ) HCUP Databases, Healthcare Cost and Utilization Project (HCUP): Overview of the Nationwide Inpatient Sample (NIS)*; 2013. Available at: http://www.hcup-us.ahrq.gov/nisoverview.jsp.

27. *Health Care Cost and Utilization Project. Introduction to the HCUP KIDS' Inpatient Database (KID), 2012*; 2016. Available at: https://hcup-us.ahrq.gov/db/nation/kid/kid_2012_introduction.jsp. Accessed July 23, 2023.

28. Medicare enrollment numbers. Center for Medicare Advocacy. Available at: https://medicareadvocacy.org/medicare-enrollment-numbers/; June 29, 2023. Accessed August 1, 2023.

29. PearlDiver, Inc.. Available at: http://www.pearldiverinc.com/.

30. https://www.ibm.com/downloads/cas/0NKLE57Y.

31. http://www.iqvia.com.

32. Poupore NS, Chidarala S, Nguyen SA, et al. Cleft lip and/or palate repair in children with hypopituitarism: analysis of the kids' inpatient database [published online ahead of print, 2022 Jul 29] *Cleft Palate Craniofac J*. 2022. https://doi.org/10.1177/10556656221117435, 10556656221117435.

33. Hanba C, Svider PF, Siegel B, et al. Pediatric thyroidectomy. *Otolaryngol Head Neck Surg*. 2017;156(2):360–367. https://doi.org/10.1177/0194599816677527.

34. Newton M, Johnson RF, Wynings E, Jaffal H, Chorney SR. Pediatric tracheostomy-related complications: a cross-sectional analysis. *Otolaryngol Head Neck Surg*. 2022;167(2):359–365. https://doi.org/10.1177/01945998211046527.

35. Hanba C, Svider PF, Lai W, et al. An investigation of operative outcomes: pediatric invasive fungal sinusitis. *Int J Pediatr Otorhinolaryngol*. 2017;102:142–147. https://doi.org/10.1016/j.ijporl.2017.09.009.

36. Lavin JM, Rusher T, Shah RK. Complications of pediatric otitis media. *Otolaryngol Head Neck Surg*. 2016;154(2):366–370. https://doi.org/10.1177/0194599815611860.

37. Choi JS, Yu J, Lovin BD, Chapel AC, Patel AJ, Gallagher KK. Effects of preoperative embolization on Juvenile nasopharyngeal angiofibroma surgical outcomes: a study of the kids' inpatient database. *J Neurol Surg B Skull Base*. 2020;83(1):76–81. https://doi.org/10.1055/s-0040-1716676. Published 2020 Oct 12.

38. Burton BN, Gilani S, Desai M, Saddawi-Konefka R, Willies-Jacobo L, Gabriel RA. Perioperative risk factors associated with morbidity and mortality following pediatric inpatient sinus surgery. *Ann Otol Rhinol Laryngol*. 2019;128(1):13–21. https://doi.org/10.1177/0003489418805504.

39. Mahairas AD, Neff R, Craker N, McNulty BN, Shinn JB, Bush ML. Trends in opioid usage following tympanoplasty and mastoidectomy. *Otol Neurotol*. 2020;41(8):e1035–e1040. https://doi.org/10.1097/MAO.0000000000002709.

40. Starr N, Oyler DR, Schadler A, Aouad RK. Chronic opioid use after laryngeal cancer treatment. *Head Neck*. 2021;43(4):1242–1251. https://doi.org/10.1002/hed.26591.

41. Massa ST, Chidambaram S, Luong P, Graboyes EM, Mazul AL. Quantifying total and out-of-pocket costs associated with head and neck cancer survivorship. *JAMA Otolaryngol Head Neck Surg.* 2022;148(12):1111−1119. https://doi.org/10.1001/jamaoto. 2022.3269.

42. Smolinski NE, Antonelli PJ, Winterstein AG. Watchful waiting for acute otitis media. *Pediatrics.* 2022;150(1):e2021055613. https://doi.org/10.1542/peds.2021-055613.

43. Eskander A, Sahovaler A, Shin J, et al. A preliminary assessment of guideline adherence and clinical variation in oral cancer treatment: a MarketScan database study. *BMC Oral Health.* 2021;21(1):270. https://doi.org/10.1186/s12903-021-01616-x. Published 2021 May 17.

44. Shokri T, Saadi R, Schaefer EW, Lighthall JG. Trends in the treatment of Bell's palsy. *Facial Plast Surg.* 2020;36(5):628−634. https://doi.org/10.1055/s-0040-1713808.

45. Jang DW, Lee HJ, Chen PG, Cohen SM, Scales CD. Management of chronic rhinosinusitis prior to otolaryngology referral: an opportunity for quality improvement. *Otolaryngol Head Neck Surg.* 2022;166(3):565−571. https://doi.org/10.1177/0194599821 1017486.

46. Brajcich BC, Fischer CP, Ko CY. Administrative and registry databases for patient safety tracking and quality improvement. *Surg Clin North Am.* 2021;101(1):121−134. https://doi.org/10.1016/j.suc.2020.09.010.

47. Campbell Jr DA, Englesbe MJ, Kubus JJ, et al. Accelerating the pace of surgical quality improvement: the power of hospital collaboration. *Arch Surg.* 2010;145(10):985−991. https://doi.org/10.1001/archsurg.2010.220.

48. Rodkey GV, Itani KM. Evaluation of healthcare quality: a tale of three giants. *Am J Surg.* 2009;198(5 Suppl):S3−S8. https://doi.org/10.1016/j.amjsurg.2009.08.004.

49. Muelleman T, Shew M, Muelleman RJ, et al. Impact of resident participation on operative time and outcomes in otologic surgery. *Otolaryngol Head Neck Surg.* 2018;158(1): 151−154. https://doi.org/10.1177/0194599817737270.

50. Feeney T, Price LL, Chen L, Graham R, Chatterjee A. Resident and fellow participation in Thyroid and Parathyroid surgery: an ACS-NSQIP clinical outcomes analysis. *J Surg Res.* 2017;220:346−352. https://doi.org/10.1016/j.jss.2017.07.030.

51. Kshirsagar RS, Chandy Z, Mahboubi H, Verma SP. Does resident involvement in thyroid surgery lead to increased postoperative complications? *Laryngoscope.* 2017;127(5): 1242−1246. https://doi.org/10.1002/lary.26176.

52. Gourishetti SC, Chen JH, Isaiah A, Vakharia K. Predictors of postoperative complications after paramedian forehead flaps. *Facial Plast Surg Aesthet Med.* 2021;23(6): 469−475. https://doi.org/10.1089/fpsam.2020.0570.

53. Katsnelson JY, Tyrell R, Karadsheh MJ, et al. Postoperative complications associated with the choice of reconstruction in head and neck cancer: an outcome analysis of 4,712 patients from the ACS-NSQIP database. *J Reconstr Microsurg.* 2022;38(5): 343−360. https://doi.org/10.1055/s-0041-1733922.

54. Panayi AC, Haug V, Kauke-Navarro M, Diehm YF, Pomahac B. The impact of metabolic syndrome on microvascular head and neck reconstruction: an ACS-NSQIP data analysis. *J Plast Reconstr Aesthetic Surg.* 2022;75(4):1360−1371. https://doi.org/10.1016/ j.bjps.2021.11.074.

55. Cheng J, Liu B, Farjat AE, Jang DW. Adverse events in endoscopic sinus surgery for infectious orbital complications of sinusitis: 30-day NSQIP pediatric outcomes. *Otolaryngol Head Neck Surg.* 2017;157(4):716−721. https://doi.org/10.1177/019459981 7717675.

56. Omiunu A, Barinsky GL, Fang CH, et al. Factors associated with unanticipated admission after outpatient endoscopic sinonasal surgery. *Laryngoscope*. 2022;132(3):518−522. https://doi.org/10.1002/lary.29687.

57. Teitelbaum JI, Grasse C, Quan D, et al. General complications after endoscopic sinus surgery in smokers: a 2005−2016 NSQIP analysis. *Ann Otol Rhinol Laryngol*. 2021;130(4):350−355. https://doi.org/10.1177/0003489420952481.

58. Mahboubi H, Haidar YM, Moshtaghi O, et al. Postoperative complications and readmission rates following surgery for cerebellopontine angle schwannomas. *Otol Neurotol*. 2016;37(9):1423−1427. https://doi.org/10.1097/MAO.0000000000001178.

59. Roxbury CR, Yang J, Salazar J, Shah RK, Boss EF. Safety and postoperative adverse events in pediatric otologic surgery: analysis of American College of Surgeons NSQIP-P 30-day outcomes. *Otolaryngol Head Neck Surg*. 2015;152(5):790−795. https://doi.org/10.1177/0194599815575711.

60. Pollei TR, Barrs DM, Hinni ML, Bansberg SF, Walter LC. Operative time and cost of resident surgical experience: effect of instituting an otolaryngology residency program. *Otolaryngol Head Neck Surg*. 2013;148(6):912−918. https://doi.org/10.1177/0194599813482291.

61. Shew MA, Muelleman T, Villwock M, et al. Therapeutic mastoidectomy does not increase postoperative complications in the management of the chronic ear. *Otol Neurotol*. 2018;39(1):54−58. https://doi.org/10.1097/MAO.0000000000001609.

62. Raghavan M, Carr M. Age and indication for pediatric septoplasty in the NSQIP-P database. *Int J Pediatr Otorhinolaryngol*. 2022;154:111046. https://doi.org/10.1016/j.ijporl.2022.111046.

63. Siddiqui AA, Favre NM, Powers K, Reese A, Carr MM. Laryngeal surgery for congenital laryngomalacia: NSQIP-P analysis of complications. *Am J Otolaryngol*. 2022;43(3):103459. https://doi.org/10.1016/j.amjoto.2022.103459.

64. American Academy of Otolaryngology−Head and Neck Surgery. Reg-ent ENT clinical data registry. Accessed Jul 23, 2023. https://www.entnet.org/quality-practice/reg-ent-clinical-data-registry/.

65. Gurgel RK, Briggs SE, Dhepyasuwan N, Rosenfeld RM. Quality improvement in otolaryngology-head and neck surgery: age-related hearing loss measures. *Otolaryngol Head Neck Surg*. 2021;165(6):765−774. https://doi.org/10.1177/01945998211000442.

66. Rizk H, Agrawal Y, Barthel S, et al. Quality improvement in Neurology: neurotology quality measurement set. *Otolaryngol Head Neck Surg*. 2018;159(4):603−607. https://doi.org/10.1177/0194599818790947.

67. Pavelchek C, Lee DS, Walia A, et al. Responsible imputation of missing speech perception testing data & analysis of 4,739 observations and predictors of performance. *Otol Neurotol*. 2023;44(6):e369−e378. https://doi.org/10.1097/MAO.0000000000003903.

68. Pavelchek C, Michelson AP, Walia A, et al. Imputation of missing values for cochlear implant candidate audiometric data and potential applications. *PLoS One*. 2023;18(2):e0281337. https://doi.org/10.1371/journal.pone.0281337. Published 2023 Feb 6.

69. Shafieibavani E, Goudey B, Kiral I, et al. Predictive models for cochlear implant outcomes: performance, generalizability, and the impact of cohort size. *Trends Hear*. 2021;25:23312165211066174. https://doi.org/10.1177/23312165211066174.

70. Barbour DL, Howard RT, Song XD, et al. Online machine learning audiometry. *Ear Hear*. 2019;40(4):918−926. https://doi.org/10.1097/AUD.0000000000000669.

71. Farrokhian N, Holcomb AJ, Dimon E, et al. Development and validation of machine learning models for predicting occult nodal metastasis in early-stage oral cavity

squamous cell carcinoma. *JAMA Netw Open*. 2022;5(4):e227226. https://doi.org/ 10.1001/jamanetworkopen.2022.7226. Published 2022 Apr 1.

72. Chowdhury NI, Smith TL, Chandra RK, Turner JH. Automated classification of osteo-meatal complex inflammation on computed tomography using convolutional neural networks. *Int Forum Allergy Rhinol*. 2019;9(1):46−52. https://doi.org/10.1002/ alr.22196.

73. Wilson BS, Tucci DL, Moses DA, et al. Harnessing the power of artificial intelligence in otolaryngology and the communication sciences. *J Assoc Res Otolaryngol*. 2022;23(3): 319−349. https://doi.org/10.1007/s10162-022-00846-2.

74. Ren J, Jing X, Wang J, et al. Automatic recognition of laryngoscopic images using a deep-learning technique. *Laryngoscope*. 2020;130(11):E686−E693. https://doi.org/ 10.1002/lary.28539.

75. Cao Z, Chen F, Grais EM, et al. Machine learning in diagnosing middle ear disorders us-ing tympanic membrane images: a meta-analysis. *Laryngoscope*. 2023;133(4):732−741. https://doi.org/10.1002/lary.30291.

76. Lesica NA. Why do hearing aids fail to restore normal auditory perception? *Trends Neurosci*. 2018;41(4):174−185. https://doi.org/10.1016/j.tins.2018.01.008.

77. Moses DA, Metzger SL, Liu JR, et al. Neuroprosthesis for decoding speech in a para-lyzed person with anarthria. *N Engl J Med*. 2021;385(3):217−227. https://doi.org/ 10.1056/NEJMoa2027540.

78. Iliadou E, Su Q, Kikidis D, Bibas T, Kloukinas C. Profiling hearing aid users through big data explainable artificial intelligence techniques. *Front Neurol*. 2022;13:933940. https:// doi.org/10.3389/fneur.2022.933940. Published 2022 Aug 26.

79. Wathour J, Govaerts PJ, Lacroix E, Naïma D. Effect of a CI programming fitting tool with artificial intelligence in experienced cochlear implant patients. *Otol Neurotol*. 2023;44(3):209−215. https://doi.org/10.1097/MAO.0000000000003810.

80. Rudman JR, Mei C, Bressler SE, Blanton SH, Liu XZ. Precision medicine in hearing loss. *J Genet Genomics*. 2018;45(2):99−109. https://doi.org/10.1016/j.jgg.2018. 02.004.

81. Shew M, New J, Wichova H, Koestler DC, Staecker H. Using machine learning to pre-dict sensorineural hearing loss based on perilymph micro RNA expression profile. *Sci Rep*. 2019;9(1):3393. https://doi.org/10.1038/s41598-019-40192-7. Published 2019 Mar 4.

82. Schmitt HA, Pich A, Prenzler NK, et al. Personalized proteomics for precision diagnos-tics in hearing loss: disease-specific analysis of human perilymph by mass spectrometry. *ACS Omega*. 2021;6(33):21241−21254. https://doi.org/10.1021/acsomega.1c01136. Published 2021 Aug 13.

83. Lin HC, Ren Y, Lysaght AC, Kao SY, Stankovic KM. Proteome of normal human peri-lymph and perilymph from people with disabling vertigo. *PLoS One*. 2019;14(6): e0218292. https://doi.org/10.1371/journal.pone.0218292. Published 2019 Jun 11.

84. Birkeland AC, Uhlmann WR, Brenner JC, Shuman AG. Getting personal: head and neck cancer management in the era of genomic medicine. *Head Neck*. 2016;38(Suppl 1): E2250−E2258. https://doi.org/10.1002/hed.24132.

85. Marret G, Bièche I, Dupain C, et al. Genomic alterations in head and neck squamous cell carcinoma: level of evidence according to ESMO scale for clinical actionability of mo-lecular targets (ESCAT). *JCO Precis Oncol*. 2021;5:215−226. https://doi.org/10.1200/ PO.20.00280.

86. https://sharing.nih.gov.

87. Thakur S, Rim TH, Ting DSJ, Hsieh YT, Kim TI. Editorial: big data and artificial intelligence in ophthalmology. *Front Med.* 2023;10:1145522. https://doi.org/10.3389/fmed.2023.1145522. Published 2023 Feb 14.

88. Eyenuk BA. A global provider of AI-powered eye screenings, scores $26m to expand reach in 18 countries. *Fierce Healthcare*; October 17, 2022. https://www.fiercehealthcare.com/ai-and-machine-learning/eyenuk-global-provider-ai-powered-eye-screenings-score-26m-series-fund. Accessed September 3, 2023.

89. Milea D, Najjar RP, Zhubo J, et al. Artificial intelligence to detect papilledema from ocular fundus photographs. *N Engl J Med.* 2020;382(18):1687−1695. https://doi.org/10.1056/NEJMoa1917130.

90. https://www.ohdsi.org/data-standardization/.

91. Saraswathula A, Roy S, Blythe WR, Gourin CG, Boss EF. The unrealized potential of the Reg-ent ENT clinical data registry [published online ahead of print, 2023 Jun 29] *JAMA Otolaryngol Head Neck Surg.* 2023. https://doi.org/10.1001/jamaoto.2023.1389, 10.1001/jamaoto.2023.1389.

92. Schmalbach CE, Brereton J, Bowman C, Denneny 3rd JC. American Academy of otolaryngology-head and neck surgery/foundation Reg-ent registry: purpose, properties, and priorities. *Otolaryngol Head Neck Surg.* 2021;164(5):964−971. https://doi.org/10.1177/0194599820984135.

Bias in big data: Historically underrepresented groups and implications

Jennifer A. Villwock, MD [1],
G. Richard Holt, MD, MSEng, MPH, MABE, MSAM, D Bioethics [2]

[1]*Professor, Otolaryngology-Head and Neck Surgery, The University of Kansas Medical Center, Kansas City, KS, United States;* [2]*Professor Emeritus, The University of Texas Health Science Center at San Antonio, San Antonio, TX, United States*

The struggle for an equitable distribution of healthcare resources in the United States has been long and unsuccessful, dating back to the founding of the country. Disparities in healthcare access and provision of equitable care remain moral and ethical challenges for the entire US healthcare industry. Meanwhile, practicing physicians, including otolaryngologists-head and neck surgeons, continue to provide the best medical care possible under these conditions. Disparities in healthcare delivery to marginalized populations and disadvantaged persons occur throughout the entire range of the system, from health policy impacts to community access.[1] Additionally, owing to the effects of global disease and health issues, increased awareness of the disparities across countries and societies has highlighted the world-wide effects of inequitable healthcare delivery which play a definite role in the acquisition of data upon which broad health policies are established.

The COVID-19 pandemic acutely brought into perspective the inadequacies of the world's healthcare delivery systems, particularly with respect to data and its analysis. Marked deficiencies existed in the acquisition of real-time data to guide the care of patients during this critical time.[2] In a time of unprecedented quantities of data—traditional medical outcomes, social media, and mobile application symptom tracking initiatives—and sophisticated analysis methods like artificial intelligence (AI) and machine learning, the system struggled to leverage this data for unbiased, evidence-based, and effective healthcare policies.

Indeed, the pandemic raised substantial awareness that much of the research data relied upon to make public health decisions was not representative of the overall population and often failed to adequately address critical components of health and disease susceptibility such as gender, ethnicity/race, socioeconomic status, social determinants of health, medical comorbidities, and other considerations. Inequities were perpetuated by the omission of underrepresented groups. This is not new in medical research. In 1977, the FDA issues a guideline banning women of childbearing age participating in clinical trials that was not formally rescinded until 1993. Generic and overly generalized data resulted in nonpersonalized care that was not effective for all patients.

This chapter will address the moral and ethical implications of inequalities and inequities in medical research with particular emphasis on how big data, machine learning, and AI must evolve to ensure appropriate inclusion of historically disadvantaged persons in the research process and in the development of the diagnostic and therapeutic algorithms upon which clinicians and patients may come to rely.

Ethical principles and big data

The four well-established principles of medical ethics include: (1) autonomy, (2) beneficence, (3) nonmaleficence, and (4) social or distributive justice. The first three principles are commonly thought of in the provision of ethical individual patient care. The fourth is of particular significance to population-based healthcare, including any endeavor employing large data. Initially interpreted as applying to the equality of distributing scarce resources in the healthcare field, the meaning of social justice has now expanded to include health equity and fairness across the range of healthcare research treatment algorithms, access to healthcare, and the identification of particular needs of populations and groups in disease prevention and treatment.

The role of big data in healthcare has become increasingly important, particularly with the recent introduction of AI and machine learning capabilities. As enthusiasm increases for AI and ML informed diagnostic and prognostic algorithms, there is real potential for inappropriate decision-making based on data that do not reflect the actual patients we see before us. Ibrahim et al. have nicely summarized these concerns, stating that "the technology-mediated transformative potential of big data is taking place within the context of historical inequities in health and health care."[3] The implications and limitations of inadequate research that has historically, and in many domains continues to, lack sufficient inclusion of marginalized groups and traditionally excluded persons. Recognition of the historical damage done to the validity of scientific and clinical data must be recognized if the advancement of evidence-based healthcare is to fulfill the requirements of medical ethics, specifically that of social or distributive justice. Healthcare disparities can be exacerbated by the unjustified exclusion of significant segments of society.

There is no shortage of groups missing within research protocols and the published literature. People from minority, minoritized, and marginalized communities have historically been excluded from research and continue to be at risk for exclusion. Much work has been done in recent years with respect to individuals identifying as belonging to minority racial and ethnic groups. The social politics of including or excluding persons of color in healthcare research is not a new phenomenon. Tong et al. posit that "race permeates clinical decision and treatment in multiple ways," indicating that providers' attitudes, data-based clinical guidelines, and stereotyping all may play a role.[4] If people from these communities are not included in the exploratory research that yields diagnostic and therapeutic recommendations, these recommendations may be fundamentally flawed when applied. This creates a moral and ethical challenge which must be addressed across the entire system of health research and care provision and is amplified as healthcare systems increasingly seek to leverage data-driven solutions. This violates the fourth principle of medical ethics—social or distributive justice.

As research studies become larger in scope and sheer volume of data collected, the data management requirements have become so complex that human oversight of the methodologies and results is no longer feasible. This has led to the rise of sophisticated techniques like AI and their applications to increasingly complex big data sets. It is important to recall that, as Norori and associates state, "Bias in the medical field can be dissected along."[5] Biased data include datasets that are not representative or fail to consider all relevant variables. It is also important to recognize that AI applications are not inherently unbiased. Even if tasked with making predictions seemingly independently, coding by humans is required in the initial humans. Leslie and colleagues authored an aptly titled commentary, "Does 'AI' stand for augmented inequality in the era of COVID-19 healthcare." They noted that bias and discrimination in design can facilitate flawed reasoning and exacerbate health inequities.[6] Biases present in these initial steps will propagate, and likely amplify, as the algorithms mature. If the conclusions and recommendations from the data mining process on biased data become healthcare guidelines, then vulnerable/marginalized populations may not be beneficiaries of the recommendations. They may also be harmed if the recommendations for healthcare are not appropriate for them. Additionally, AI does not consider how the conclusions drawn from its analyses may affect human beings. There are no checks and balances to ensure that outputs are relevant and appropriate given specific clinical or cultural contexts. Resultant algorithms can be the drivers of practice guidelines for clinicians, as well as potentially encoded in patient care requirements in electronic health records. If the data input has no basis in medical ethics, the eventual output will be ethics-free, as well. After all, equity, diversity, access, fairness and transparency, and accuracy of data applied to patient care are all ethical constructs. Machines cannot be expected to make ethical decisions, so humans must provide vigilant oversight.

Biases and missing data concerns in big data studies

The desire for "clean" data that can be analyzed with a minimum of confounding factors drives study inclusion and exclusion criteria. However, while these simplified cohorts of study participants may facilitate data analysis, they are unlikely to reflect to population at large. This limits the external validity of results and perpetuates exclusions (or discrimination). Whatever the reason, "structural inequalities, biases, and racism in society are easily encoded in datasets."[7] Table 6.1 provides examples

Table 6.1 Categories of missing persons in research studies.

Category	Examples of missing people	% US population
Race	Racial and/or ethnic minorities.	24.5%
Age	People above a certain age threshold without scientific justification for exclusion (e.g., > 65 years old).	16.8%
Ability	People with physical disabilities may be excluded despite lack of foundational clinical data upon which to gauge their suitability for a particular study	13%
Mental health		20%
Military service	Veterans may have experienced unique toxic or traumatic exposures, which result in their exclusion from studies.	6.4%
Geography	Urban and rural patients may face unique challenges in both presenting for care and participating in research studies and may be excluded by default as a result.	
Social determinants of health	Factors such as health literacy, relationship with the healthcare system, access to care, experience of discrimination in the community, and/or healthcare setting may adversely impact both likelihood to participate in research and access to care.	
Language	Nonnative speakers of English who speak English less than "very well" may be excluded for no other reason than lack of translated materials and study methods into their preferred language.	8.3%
Sex and gender	Women were historically excluded from clinical trials. Men may be excluded from research on female predominant pathologies such as breast cancer.	51.1% (women)
	Recognition of gender identity beyond the traditional male or female dichotomy may complicate categorization and analysis of data from individuals whose gender is not the same as their sex.	5% young adults identify as transgender or nonbinary

of common categories of exclusion. It is important to note that excluding people from these categories may not be intentional. For example, large clinical trials historically struggle to enroll representative proportions of racial and ethnic minorities. This may be due to lack of trust in clinical research due to historic abuses, insufficient outreach to these communities, or other factors. However, these reasons are insufficient to justify continuing this status quo and dedicated efforts must be made to rectify these issues.

While harmful racial biases have received the bulk of attention and recognition that they are harmful to the health of a significant sector of the US population, concern must also be raised for biases of gender, age, disability, mental health, and other conditions that can be unequally addressed in large population studies and big data analyses. When viewed from the broader lens of discrimination, the needs of people belonging to these groups must also be recognized as potentially marginalized and disregarded. Gender plays a role in the biological definitions of health and wellness, as well as in response to disease and disease treatment. For decades, research studies on heart disease in females were largely disregarded, yet it is one of the leading causes of death and disability in women. Breast cancer in males, although a small percentage of the overall population with the disease, is not the same cancer as in women. Treatment extrapolated from studies in women is not entirely appropriate. Older and elderly persons may be excluded from participating in large-scale research protocols owing to their comorbidities and increased risks for side effects of the study arms. Currently, with gender polarity under change, accommodations must be made for those who do not identify with their biological designation. Persons with physical disabilities may be excluded from research studies as well, and this exclusion (or discrimination) may be perpetuated over the years by a lack of foundational clinical data upon which to gauge their suitability for a particular study. Inclusion of disabled persons requires thoughtful consideration, as well as a fundamental understanding of the uniqueness of disabled persons.[8] Millions of Americans live with disabling conditions in the US, yet their impairment does not necessarily negate their participation in a general population study. People with disabilities also suffer from common population disorders—heart disease, colon cancer, pulmonary disease—and they deserve to be included in appropriate studies. While this may complicate study design and how to divide participants into cohorts for data analysis, valuable health data can, and should, still be obtained from these groups to inform the results of the health issue under study. Timmons et al. commented that "AI applications will not mitigate mental health disparities if they are built from historical data that reflect underlying social biases and inequities."[9] As with persons with disabilities, those with mental health disorders may not be considered as potential study volunteers and excluded from a study that could provide valuable information on a common health condition found in both those with and without mental health disorders. The stigmata of mental health disorders may detrimentally exclude otherwise reasonable study candidates from being considered for participation.

When considered through the lens of the ethical principle of social/distributive justice, there is an obligation to intentionally include historically marginalized and excluded persons in medical research. Ford and colleagues, in a systematic review of the barriers to underrepresented populations' participation in cancer trials, stated that "racial and ethnic minorities, older adults, rural residents, and individuals of low socioeconomic stats are underrepresented among participants in cancer-related trials."[10] Similarly, Spector-Bagdady et al. conducted a retrospective study of patients to explore how recruitment techniques affected the diversity of participants in a research data bank. They found that "compared with the overall clinical population, patients who consented to enroll in the research data bank were significantly less diverse in terms of age, sex, race, ethnicity, and socioeconomic status."[11] Awareness, opportunity, and acceptance of participation have been identified as key determinants of participation. Thoughtful interventions to reduce the disparities in clinical trials and research data banks are needed. The same is needed in big data studies to avoid skewed conclusions that may be further detrimental to the health of those already marginalized in healthcare.

In our increasingly global society—including things like datasets and public health information from countries with nationalized healthcare—it is important to recognize that marginalized populations exist internationally and suffer from the same exclusionary practices previously mentioned. Additionally, these factors may be exacerbated by poverty, lack of resources, or researchers' lack of appropriate cultural context for interpreting data analysis results. Wesson and colleagues addressed the issue of ensuring equity in the application of big data research in public health, identifying that social and environmental determinants are important in providing the best available intervention.[12] The medical and scientific communities have an ethical obligation to utilize the powers of AI and machine learning in the amalgamation of global health data for the purpose of better understanding the health needs of low-income countries and the development of innovations in healthcare that fit the needs of that specific population in a resource and culturally appropriate manner.

Addressing the problem

Since computer systems, especially AI systems, do not yet have ethical and morality capabilities, we cannot rely on them to apply medical ethics. Rather, healthcare professionals must shoulder the responsibility for providing context and oversight to the systems that gather, analyze, and draw conclusions from big data. This involves vigilance and effort to alleviate the harmful biases that propagate into the systems from historical data—and historical approaches to subject recruitment and data collection—and developing countermeasures to prevent harm to vulnerable populations not well represented in the raw data (Table 6.2).

While there are ethical considerations and safeguards that must be put into place regarding big data and AI applications, it is important to remember the enormous potential of these technologies. Significant positive outcomes from big data analyses can inform clinical care, improve diagnostic and therapeutic innovations, and make healthcare delivery systems more accessible and efficient. Rajkomar and colleagues posit that rather than simply guarding against healthcare harms posed by machine learning models, the systems should be used to advance health equity.[13]

The ethical principle of distributive (social) justice should be incorporated throughout the entire process, beginning with the design, to ensure that the models benefit all patients without bias. Clinicians must use their professional judgment

Table 6.2 Common problems in big data ethics and their mitigation.

Ethical problems in big data	Potential mitigative actions
Limited scientific data/studies	Identify and support national and global studies that include underrepresented populations
Lack of high power tools to identify ethical issues in research involving big data	Develop major mandates in science and medicine to employ artificial intelligence and machine learning to query studies for ethical conduct based on appropriate guidelines
Lack of consensus on ethical concerns in the use of big data	Develop ethical guidelines for big data studies that can mandate compliance
Absence of strong central and point of study ethical oversight	National legislation for the formation of big data ethical oversight entities
Absence of commercial big data regulations for ethical design of proprietary studies	Federal regulations for the proper inclusion of ethical review of proprietary big data studies

when reviewing practice guidelines that have the potential for marginalizing certain populations that have been characteristically absent from critical retrospective and prospective studies. New strategies need to be developed that may be more successful in the recruitment and enrollment process for diversity. As Dr. Joan Teno, noted in JAMA Health Forum about the use of big data in medical practice, "garbage in, garbage out."[14] If big data practice guidelines built from AI algorithms are to be applied ethically and equitably to diverse populations in the US—and globally—the evidence supporting the guidelines must also be ethical and equitable as well.

Another focus for improvement is at the level of the engineers who design and develop the protocols and algorithms for big data analyses. Increasing the diversity of this group of computer and systems engineers could intentionally improve awareness of the issues of inclusivity and equality/equity in data input and analyses. Further, linking physician researchers with the design engineers could provide a more medically professional approach to the reduction of intrinsic and extrinsic biases, as well as introducing the concepts of biomedical ethics into the system design.

There is also a need for more healthcare researchers and physicians, even if not directly involved in big data research, to obtain a minimum level of literacy in these topics. This will help ensure appropriate vetting of scientific articles occurs during peer review. These scientific reviewers are the first line of defense to ensure that inclusion criteria were not overly restrictive and sufficient diversity is present in the sample; that appropriate analyses were undertaken; and that results are interpreted in the proper clinical, societal, and cultural contexts. Without baseline big data literacy, it is easy to be impressed and distracted by large sample numbers and small P-values, which may belie overreaching or ungeneralizable conclusions.

Additional oversight will need to come from institutional review boards (IRBs) and other institutional oversight mechanisms as well as the input of the community of those who have characteristically been marginalized and biased against. Moon and colleagues recognize that "the essential conflict in research is the duty to avoid allowing the ends to justify the means," which has been the rationale of many of the worst examples of inhumane research in the world.[15] If researchers have difficulties understanding how their research protocol design may disadvantage certain persons or groups, or lend greater advantage to others, then it falls to the IRB to provide the ethical conscience on behalf of the potential subjects. Research ethics reflects clinical ethics in many respects, including respect for persons (autonomy and nonmaleficence), beneficence, and social/distributive justice.

In conclusion, big data, AI, and machine learning are potentially unique and positive innovations to medical science, with the capability of analyzing tremendous amounts of data and providing mechanistic insights into health data impressions and potential salutary clinical pathways. But these are not humanistic, nor are they capable of considering ethics and morality in their analysis of data, no matter how large the data set is. For now, humans are better at understanding humans than machines. Thus, the ultimate responsibility for ensuring that clinical outcomes data are appropriate rests with clinicians and ethical researchers. The data input must be based on the broad demographics of our society, reflect the ethics and morality of the healthcare profession, and meet the needs of the population, including, and especially, those who are historically marginalized and disregarded.

References

1. Hamed S, Bradby H, Ahlberg BM, et al. Racism in healthcare: a scoping review. *BMC Publ Health*. 2022;22:988. https://doi.org/10.1186/s12889-022-13122-y.
2. Yearby R, Clark B, Figueroa JF. Structural racism in historical and modern US health care policy. *Health Aff*. 2022;41(2):187–194. https://doi.org/10.1377/hlthaff.2021.01466.
3. Ibrahim SA, Charlson ME, Neill DB. Big data analytics and the struggle for equity in health care: the promise and perils. *Health Equity*. April 1, 2020;4(1):99–101. https://doi.org/10.1089/heq.2019.0112.
4. Tong M, Artiga S. Use of race in clinical diagnosis and decision-makiing: overview and implications. *Kaiser Family Found*. 2021;9. https://www.kff.org/report-section/use-of-race-in-clinical-diagnosis-and-decision-making-overview-and-implications-issue-brief/.
5. Norori N, Hu Q, Aellen FM, Faraci FD, Tzovara A. Addressing bias in big data and AI for health care: a call for open science. *Patterns (N Y)*. October 8, 2021;2(10):100347. https://doi.org/10.1016/j.patter.2021.100347.
6. Leslie D, Mazumder A, Peppin A, Wolters MK, Hagerty A. Does "AI" stand for augmenting inequality in the era of covid-19 healthcare? *BMJ*. 2021;372:n304. https://doi.org/10.1136/bmj.n304.

7. Knight HE, Keeny SR, Dreyer K, et al. Challenging racism in the use of health data. *Lancet Digit Health*. 2021;3(3):E144−E146. https://doi.org/10.1016/S2589-7500(21) 00019-4.

8. Wald M. AI data-driven personalization and disability inclusion. *Front Artif Intell*. 2021; 5:571955. https://doi.org/10.3389/frai.2020.571955.

9. Timmons AC, Duong JB, Simo Fiallo N, et al. A call to action on assessing and mitigating bias. Artificial intelligence applications for mental health. *Perspect Psychol Sci*. 2022;18. https://doi.org/10.1177/17456916221134490.

10. Ford JG, Howerton MW, Lai GY, et al. Barriers to recruiting underrepresented populations to cancer clinical trials: a systematic review. *Cancer*. January 15, 2008;112(2): 228−242. https://doi.org/10.1002/cncr.23157.

11. Spetor-Badady K, Tang S, Jabour S, et al. Respecting autonomy and enabling diversity: the effect of eligibility and enrollment on research data. *Health Aff*. 2021;40(12): 1892−1899. https://doi.org/10.1377/hlthaff.2021.01197.

12. Wesson P, Hswen Y, Valdes G, Stojanovski K, Handley MA. Risks and opportunities to ensure equity in the application of big data research in public health. *Annu Rev Publ Health*. April 2022;43:59−78. https://doi.org/10.1146/annurev-publhealth-051920- 110928.

13. Rajkomar A, Hardt M, Howell MD, Corrado G, Chin MH. Ensuring fairness in machine learning to advance health equity. *Ann Intern Med*. December 18, 2018;169(12): 866−872. https://doi.org/10.7326/M18-1990.

14. Teno JM. Garbage in, garbage out–words of caution on big data and machine learning in medical practice. *JAMA Health Forum*. February 3, 2023;4(2):e230397. https://doi.org/ 10.1001/jamahealthforum.2023.0397.

15. Moon MR, Khin-Maung-Gyi F. The history and role of institutional review boards. *Virt Mentor*. 2009;11(4):311−321. https://doi.org/10.1001/virtualmentor.2009.11.4.pfor1- 0904.

Further reading

1. Arcaya MC, Arcaya AL, Subramanian SV. Inequalities in health: definitions, concepts, and theories. *Glob Health Action*. June 24, 2015;8:27106. https://doi.org/10.3402/ gha.v8.27106.

2. McCallum JM, Arekere DM, Green BL, Katz RV, Rivers BM. Awareness and knowledge of the U.S. Public Health Service syphilis study at Tuskegee: implications for biomedical research. *J Health Care Poor Underserved*. November 2006;17(4):716−733. https:// doi.org/10.1353/hpu.2006.0130.

3. Ntoutsi E, Fafalios P, Gadiraju U, et al. Bias in data-driven artificial intelligence systems—an introductory survey. *WIREs Data Min Knowl Discov*. 2020;10:e1356. https://doi.org/10.1002/widm.1356.

Artificial intelligence in otolaryngology

7

Nathan Farrokhian, MD, Andrés M. Bur, MD, FACS, Associate Professor

Department of Otolaryngology—Head and Neck Surgery, University of Kansas,
Kansas City, KS, United States

Introduction

Otolaryngologists, like other medical practitioners, routinely face the question, "Should I operate on this patient?" The decision-making process for such a question is complex. Patients exhibit considerable variability, and surgical outcomes are not universally successful. Consequently, clinicians rely on heuristic models informed by similar patients rather than searching for an identical patient in a textbook or case report. These heuristic models are primarily derived from the statistical analysis of aggregated patient outcomes.

Statistics encompasses a set of techniques used to analyze, interpret, and draw conclusions from data. These techniques have become the cornerstone of evidence-based clinical medicine. Most clinicians are proficient at interpreting basic statistical models and incorporating their findings into daily clinical practice. However, statistical models impose rigid assumptions about the underlying probability distribution of the data and necessitate a priori knowledge of variable relationships. For instance, linear regression assumes a linear relationship between each input variable and the desired output, while logistic regression assumes a logarithmic relationship between variable values and the probability of a binary outcome. When the true underlying variable relationships deviate from these assumptions, the model fit becomes inefficient, and prediction accuracy decreases.

In the context of human diseases, patient variables seldom adhere to these rigid assumptions. Moreover, clinicians often lack complete insight into the specific variables driving outcomes and are subject to cognitive bias. Patient variables frequently exhibit high dependence, and in the case of radiographical imaging, they can even be imperceptible to the human eye. This is where artificial intelligence (AI) models demonstrate significant potential to revolutionize clinical practice. In recent years, there has been a surge of interest in AI applications across all medical disciplines, with some already being integrated into clinical practice. IDx-DR, the first US Food and Drug Administration (FDA)-approved AI model in the USA, is a deep learning algorithm that diagnoses diabetic retinopathy from retinal images with such high accuracy that physician interpretation is unnecessary. Another example, Karius, employs machine learning algorithms to rapidly analyze microbial cell-

Big Data in Otolaryngology. https://doi.org/10.1016/B978-0-443-10520-3.00005-8

free DNA isolated from plasma samples to provide infectious etiological diagnoses. These examples represent only a fraction of the recently developed models using radiological, pathological, and clinical data that are being incorporated into daily clinical practice.

Historically, AI conjured images of talking machines and robot companions. While these ideas are not entirely unfounded, especially with the rapidly increasing quality of large language models (LLMs), most real-world AI applications focus on driving practical advancements in everyday tasks. This chapter introduces the fundamental concepts of AI and their application to the clinical practice of otolaryngology.

Fundamentals of artificial intelligence

AI models encompass a wide range of algorithms capable of learning and adapting their rule set without being explicitly programmed (e.g., "hard coded"). These models range from simple filters, such as those that recognize spam emails, to more complex systems that make real-time decisions in moving vehicles. At their core, AI models aim to learn complex relationships between variables to generate predictions based on specific input data. This adaptability enables the development of flexible and effective solutions to a broad array of tasks across various disciplines, including otolaryngology. AI algorithms utilize input data to generate specific outputs, which can be binary (e.g., "cancer" or "no cancer"), multioutput, or even the synthesis of images, speech, or video. For instance, an AI model might generate a risk score for a particular medical condition based on a patient's medical history and demographic information.

Traditional machine learning models

Traditional machine learning models, often considered the simplest form of AI algorithms, are characterized by the structure of their input data.

In **supervised learning models**, the algorithm is provided with the correct output for each set of inputs during training. A model can be trained on clinicopathological variables from patients with known clinical endpoints, such as the presence of subclinical nodal metastatic disease. The algorithm then optimizes prediction of this endpoint by identifying patterns in the input data that minimize error and result in the best predictive performance. Once trained, this model can be applied to new patients as a risk assessment tool to guide the need for elective neck dissection, improving the quality and efficiency of surgical decision-making.

Unsupervised models are not provided with any output data and are thus blinded to any subgroups or labels associated with the inputs. Consequently, these models aim to find underlying patterns or structure inherent to the input data. An example of this would be the clustering of mRNA expression data from tumor samples, which could be helpful in identifying different tumor subtypes. While these tumors could all appear morphologically similar on traditional histopathological evaluation, clustering based on their mRNA expression profiles could reveal subtypes associated with higher propensity for metastatic spread or treatment resistance.

Reinforcement learning models interact with an environment and receive quantitative feedback based on this interaction. These models iteratively adapt their interactions to maximize their cumulative reward through trial and error. For example, dosing optimization in patients with chronic diseases can be modeled as a Markov decision process (MDP). In this scenario, the state of a diabetic patient can be represented by their clinicodemographic variables, including their current plasma glucose value. The model interacts with this state through an insulin dose recommendation and receives quantitative feedback that rewards plasma glucose within the goal range and punishes deviations from this range. Subsequent dosing recommendations are adjusted accordingly.

A major limitation of traditional machine learning models is the need to explicitly define the input data, often through manual feature engineering, prior to model development. In medicine, this is feasible for discrete clinical or demographic data, but integrating high-dimensional data sources such as radiographic studies, histopathologic images, or genomic data is often not practical or achievable.

Artificial neural networks

Artificial neural networks (ANNs) were specifically designed to handle complex, high-dimensional input data. Inspired by the structure and physiology of the human nervous system, ANNs consist of a collection of interconnected nodes. Similar to the summation of excitatory and inhibitory postsynaptic potentials at the axon hillock, a node receives the weighted sum of inputs from other nodes and uses an activation function to output a nonlinear transformation of its input. These nodes are organized into layers, with each layer assigned a specific function within the network. Commonly, these are organized into input, hidden, and output layers.

The input layer serves as the initial interface between the input data and the neural network. Traditionally, no calculations or transformations are performed on the data within this layer. Each node contained within this layer represents a single input feature, or variable. In clinical medicine, there could be a node corresponding to age, BMI, or even the nucleotide sequence at a specific gene locus.

The data are then passed from this input layer to the hidden layers of the network. Nodes within hidden layers utilize activation functions to perform nonlinear transformations of the input data. This allows the network to gradually learn complex representations of the input data. For example, when processing radiographical imaging data, one hidden layer might learn to represent geometrical shapes, while another layer may represent the texture features of the image. The representation learned within each hidden layer is not explicitly assigned, but rather learned via a process known as backpropagation, wherein the assigned weights of nodal connections are iteratively calibrated to minimize output error. This iterative process allows for increasingly complex, multidimensional representations, such as combinations of anatomical locations, geometric shapes, and textures that are indicative of a particular disease.

The output layer translates the information learned by the hidden layers into a format suitable for the specific task, such as a probability distribution for classification tasks or a multidimensional parameter space for generative image tasks. The true value of these models is realized here. Humans are limited by their perceptual abilities and cognitive capacity. Most diagnostic and prognostic criteria are purposefully simplified to cater to these biological limitations, which in turn improves their understandability. The rise of AI models and the associated movement away from this reductionistic perspective in medicine is discussed later in this chapter.

Deep learning models

Deep learning models are a subset of ANNs with many hidden layers, enabling them to learn even more complex representations of the input data.

Convolutional neural networks (CNNs), for instance, are specifically designed to process images and other grid-like data structures (e.g., videos and volumetric data). What makes CNNs unique is their ability to exploit the spatial structure of the data through implementation of convolutional layers. These layers perform local operations on small, overlapping regions of the input, allowing the model to capture local patterns, such as edges, corners, and textures. This property enables CNNs to learn translation-invariant features, meaning that they can recognize patterns regardless of their position in the input image. Additionally, CNNs employ pooling layers to reduce the spatial dimensions of the input, promoting translation invariance and computational efficiency. The combination of these properties makes CNNs exceptionally well suited for image-based medical tasks, such as the analysis of endoscopic images, head and neck radiology, and histopathological slides.

Recurrent neural networks (RNNs) are designed to handle sequential data, such as time series or natural language. The unique property of RNNs lies in their ability to maintain an internal state or "memory" that captures information from previous time steps in the sequence. This allows RNNs to process sequences of varying lengths and learn long-range dependencies between elements in the sequence. Consequently, RNNs are well suited for tasks where the order of the input data matters, such as processing electronic health records, dynamic treatment optimization, and natural language processing.

Ensemble learning

Modular neural networks (MNNs), also known as ensemble learning or committee machines, are a type of ANN architecture that combines multiple smaller networks to form a larger, more complex network. The unique property of MNNs is their ability to divide a complex problem into smaller, more manageable subproblems, with each module or subnetwork responsible for learning a specific aspect of the problem.

The outputs of these subnetworks are then combined, typically through methods such as voting, averaging, or weighted summation, to produce a final output.

The modular approach offers several advantages, including improved generalization, faster learning, and greater robustness to noisy data. In otolaryngology, MNNs can be applied to tasks that involve multiple data sources or require the integration of various types of information. For example, an MNN could be used to predict the risk of postoperative complications by combining information from preoperative imaging, laboratory tests, and clinical notes. Another application could be the detection of voice disorders, where an MNN can simultaneously analyze acoustic, physiological, and perceptual features to improve discrimination of neurological disorders associated with dysphonia.

Interpreting artificial intelligence models

The quality of most machine learning algorithms is evaluated using well-established performance metrics. Commonly used metrics include accuracy, precision, recall, specificity, F1 score, and area under the receiver operating characteristic curve (AUC-ROC) (Table 7.1). These metrics help clinicians assess the reliability and utility of the developed models.

Area under the receiver operating characteristic curve

Arguably the most important metric for clinical applications of AI is the AUC-ROC. This popular performance metric evaluates a model's ability to discriminate between two classes or outcomes. In the context of otolaryngology, this could involve distinguishing between patients with and without a specific disease or predicting a binary outcome, such as the success or failure of a surgical intervention.

Understanding the AUC-ROC necessitates familiarity with the receiver operating characteristic (ROC) curve, which is a graphical representation of the trade-off between a model's true positive rate (sensitivity) and false positive rate (1-specificity) at various probability thresholds. The true positive rate measures the proportion of actual positive cases that are correctly identified by the model, while the false positive rate measures the proportion of actual negative cases that are incorrectly identified as positive.

A higher AUC-ROC value (closer to 1) indicates better discrimination ability of the model, whereas an AUC-ROC value of 0.5 suggests that the model performs no better than random chance. In clinical settings, a higher AUC-ROC is desirable as it demonstrates the model's ability to effectively classify patients based on their disease status or predict other binary outcomes.

Interpreting an ROC curve:

- An ideal ROC curve has the majority of its points along the top-left corner of the graph. This area corresponds to model performance where the true positive rate

Table 7.1 Common performance metrics to assess quality of machine learning algorithms.

Metric	Definition	Formula/Calculation	Interpretation
Accuracy	The proportion of correct predictions made by the model out of the total number of predictions.	(TP + TN)/(TP + TN + FP + FN)	A higher accuracy indicates better performance. However, accuracy may not be a good metric when the class distribution is imbalanced, as the model may perform poorly on the minority class but still achieve high overall accuracy.
Precision	The proportion of true positive predictions out of all positive predictions made by the model.	TP/(TP + FP)	Precision is a measure of how many of the positively predicted instances are actually positive. A higher precision means fewer false positives. In clinical settings, high precision is desirable when the cost of a false positive is high, such as when very morbid treatments are involved.
Recall (sensitivity)	The proportion of true positive predictions out of all actual positive instances.	TP/(TP + FN)	Recall is a measure of how well the model can identify positive instances. A higher recall means fewer false negatives. In clinical settings, high recall is desirable when the cost of a false negative is high, such as when missing a serious condition can lead to severe consequences for the patient.
Specificity	The proportion of true negative predictions out of all actual negative instances.	TN/(TN + FP)	Specificity is a measure of how well the model can identify negative instances. A higher specificity means fewer false positives. In clinical settings, high specificity is desirable when it is important to accurately rule out a condition, minimizing unnecessary follow-up tests or treatments.
F1 score	The harmonic mean of precision and recall, providing a single metric to evaluate the trade-off between precision and recall.	2 * (precision * recall)/(precision + recall)	The F1 score ranges from 0 to 1, with a higher score indicating better performance. It is a useful metric when there is an uneven class distribution or when both false positives and false negatives are important to consider, as it seeks a balance between precision and recall.
AUC-ROC	The area under the receiver operating characteristic (ROC) curve, which plots the true positive rate (sensitivity) against the false positive rate (1-specificity) for various threshold settings.	N/A	The AUC-ROC ranges from 0 to 1, with a higher value indicating better performance. A model with an AUC-ROC of 0.5 is equivalent to random guessing, while a value of 1 represents perfect classification. AUC-ROC is a useful metric for evaluating the performance of a model across a range of decision thresholds and is less sensitive to class imbalance than accuracy. It provides a single measure of the model's ability to discriminate between positive and negative instances. In otolaryngology, an AUC-ROC close to 1 for a diagnostic model indicates excellent performance in differentiating between patients with and without a specific condition, such as head and neck cancer or hearing loss.

is high and the false positive rate is low, indicating effective discrimination between positive and negative cases.

- The area under the ROC curve, or AUC-ROC, is an indicator of overall model performance. As a rule of thumb, an AUC-ROC value above 0.9 is considered excellent, between 0.8 and 0.9 is considered good, between 0.7 and 0.8 is considered fair, between 0.6 and 0.7 is considered poor, and below 0.6 is considered noninformative.
- The optimal threshold on the ROC curve represents the point along the curve where the trade-off between the true positive rate and false positive rate is optimal for a specific clinical application. This threshold will depend on the relative importance of minimizing false positives versus false negatives.

AI in medicine: General applications and commonly used terms

Clinical decision support systems

Broadly, a decision support system (DSS) is a digital information system designed to improve the efficiency and accuracy of complex decisions. At their core, these systems integrate data from multiple sources and synthesize these data to identify actionable insights that are subsequently presented to the user. This acts to streamline the decision-making process, which in turn promotes decisions that are timely, informed, and efficient.

Since the advent of the electronic medical record (EMR), **clinical decision support systems (CDSSs)** have become an integral part of patient care. These systems help clinicians quickly gleam insights from the vast information contained within a patient's medical record. In the outpatient setting, most EMRs have the capability to cross-reference simple demographic information with well-established primary and secondary prevention guidelines to prompt orders for past due vaccinations and screening tests. In the inpatient setting, vital signs can be analyzed in real time to quickly risk stratify patients for sepsis, severe sepsis, and septic shock. Once identified, suggested work-up and management plans are presented to the clinician, resulting in more rapid initiation of treatment and improving outcomes in these patients.[1,2]

Given the ever-increasing complexity of predictive models, automated data curation and synthesis from the EMR will continue to improve, supporting the clinical application of these models. With the advent of LLMs, unstructured data (e.g., free text notes) have already become more readily indexed and queried. Leveraging the EMR as a data repository via CDSS will help to better integrate downstream AI-based models to assist clinicians in diagnosing complex cases, optimizing treatment strategies, and predicting patient outcomes, serving as valuable adjuncts to traditional clinical decision-making, improving the quality and efficiency of care delivery.

From reductionism to "omics": Genomics, transcriptomics, radiomics

Driven predominantly by practical imperatives, clinical medicine has been heavily reliant on a reductionistic perspective. Human cognition is inherently limited in its computational capacity, which in turn necessitated the development of heuristic models that have allowed physicians to quickly make decisions from a narrow range of data. Advancements in analytic techniques have been paralleled with increased data curation of large-scale and high-dimensional datasets. Evidence that more comprehensive datasets can provide improved outcomes via more accurate diagnostics and prognostication has ushered in a new era of clinical decision-making.

While lacking a clear etymological origin, the suffix "-omic" has come to be defined as "wholeness," "the entirety of a class," or "a study of the totality." These disciplines focus on the collective characterization and quantification of all relevant subunits that define a particular field.

Genomics, one of the original entrants to this space, focuses on precise mapping of the genetic blueprint that defines each organism. Similar to ingredients in a recipe, an individual's genetic profile defines them at the molecular level. Transcriptomics takes a step beyond genetic coding, focusing on gene expression profiles under various physiological and pathological conditions. Study of this more dynamic process offers insight into how intricacies at the genetic level interact to produce specific phenotypes; a key to understanding individualized differences in disease susceptibility and response to treatment.

Radiomics is an emerging field that involves the high-throughput extraction of quantitative features from radiological images, converting these images into minable data. By quantifying patterns, textures, and features, radiomics can detect information about disease-specific processes that are imperceptible to the human eye and thus not accessible through traditional visual inspection of images. These subvisual features have been shown to be valuable for diagnosis, predicting response to treatment and risk assessment of many diseases.

These are only a select few examples from a much greater collection of fields. The reductionist lens once showed a world in black and white, but the 'omics lens contains the entire spectrum of colors. This signifies a pivotal paradigm shift in modern medicine: a movement away from attributing diseases to individual, isolated factors and, instead, toward a comprehensive, multilayered understanding of disease.

Personalized medicine: A paradigm shift from algorithmic medicine

Personalized medicine, also referred to as precision medicine, emphasizes tailoring medical decisions, treatments, and interventions to characteristics unique to each patient. This revolution has been primarily fueled by technological advancements in 'omics and more powerful data analytics, enabling improved and more consistent resolution of individual variability.

Historically, medical decision-making has relied heavily on generalized algorithms. Given incomplete understanding and previous inability to reliably measure individual variability, large-scale clinical trials have pooled data from diverse patient groups to "wash-out" interpatient variability and determine one-size-fits-all treatment regimens. While algorithmic medicine provided a foundational approach to standardized care, the future of medicine is undeniably personalized. Instead of adhering to rigid decision thresholds, personalized medicine embraces individual nuances by leveraging an integrated, multifaceted data approach to generate patient-centric, tailored interventions. The innate parametric laxity of AI models makes them perfectly suited for these tasks.

Applications of AI in otolaryngology
Head and neck cancer

The landscape of head and neck cancer care is rapidly evolving, with AI emerging as a powerful catalyst in driving transformative changes. AI's influence doesn't merely introduce new methods; it amplifies and refines existing protocols, with the goal of improving patient outcomes across the entire care spectrum. From initial phases of diagnosis to the intricate nuances of treatment planning, prognosis, and vigilant monitoring of recurrence, AI has unfurled new avenues to augment and refine oncology care delivery.

Innovatively dubbed as "optical biopsy," recent advancements in optical imaging modalities have revolutionized how we approach cancer risk assessment. These modalities can now swiftly evaluate suspicious lesions, strategically guide biopsy procedures, and, in real-time, assist with intraoperative margin assessment.[3–6] This technology shows promise to reduce biopsy errors and improve clearance of primary malignancies at time of definitive surgical extirpation. The implications are profound as this is not just a leap in diagnostic and surgical precision; it signifies a broader horizon for head and neck cancer screenings, especially in resource-limited environments.

When delving into the realm of data-driven models, the picture becomes even more compelling. Even those models constructed purely from clinicodemographic data have demonstrated their mettle in treatment planning[7–9] and posttreatment prognostication.[10–12]

Integration of radiomics data further sharpens the predictive power of these models. With the ability to extract and integrate subvisual features, AI elucidates nuances previously imperceivable to the human eye. From initial patient interactions and work-up, these models integrate pretreatment data to aid in risk stratification,[13–16] pinpointing local high-risk features, and discerning potential regional metastases.[17–19] Its potential extends to the automated diagnosis of thyroid nodules simply from ultrasound images[20] and, importantly, in forecasting treatment responses, laying the foundation for future adaptive clinical trial protocols.[21,22]

Remarkably, many of these models have surpassed the performance of traditional AJCC TNM risk stratification benchmarks.

AI algorithms can assist in treatment planning by predicting the optimal treatment modalities for individual patients, demonstrating potential to improve patient outcomes and reduce healthcare costs. Specifically, models have been developed that are capable of analyzing imaging and dosimetric data, enabling the automated segmentation of target volumes and organs at risk,[23–27] optimization of dose distributions,[28–31] and even automated identification of contouring errors.[32] Interestingly, these often outperform manual delineation in terms of consistency and efficiency without compromising accuracy. Additionally, machine learning-guided insights in adjuvant treatment planning have shown promise in accurately identifying candidates for treatment escalation or de-escalation, which could reduce recurrence and decrease unnecessary treatment related toxicities.[33,34]

In a similar vein, generative algorithms have emerged with the novel capability of synthesizing high-resolution computed tomography (CT) images from magnetic resonance imaging (MRI) sequences[35,36] and even low-resolution daily cone beam CT scans,[37] with the latter having tremendous implications for midtreatment radiotherapy adjustments and fine-tuning adaptive dose optimization.[38]

Through the lens of AI, automated classification systems can discern gross tumor specimens,[39] delineate margins on surgical specimens,[40] and determine pathologic diagnosis from histopathological slide images.[41–43] Detection of HPV directly from standard hematoxylin and eosin (H&E) stained slides is an exemplar of AI's microscopic prowess, outperforming board-certified pathologists.[44] Beyond merely identifying structures and cells, models have been developed to quantify cellular differentiation patterns,[45] intricately map the tumor microenvironment,[46] and translate these features into actionable prognostic implications.[47]

Voice

As a foundational level, the utility of AI in voice assessment is evident in models capable of reliably differentiating between normal and pathologic voice samples.[48,49] AI-driven systems have even demonstrated improved consistency to the GRBAS scale scoring, reducing the variability traditionally seen in human interpretation.[50] Multioutput algorithms have shown that further granularity in diagnosis is possible with accurate differentiation of conditions such as hyperkinetic dysphonia, hypokinetic dysphonia, and reflux laryngitis.[51] This has been further extended to differentiate between an even wider range of laryngeal pathologies including vocal atrophy, unilateral vocal paralysis, vocal fold polyps, polypoid corditis, and adductor spasmodic dysphonia prior to laryngoscopic examination.[52,53] Similar to the aforementioned optical biopsy, image classifiers have been built that outperform physicians at identifying laryngeal neoplasms from laryngoscopy findings[54] and can even diagnose laryngeal disorders from high-speed videoendoscopy examinations.[55,56] Moreover, AI's potential as a diagnostic adjunct for conditions like Parkinson's disease, using voice as an indicator, is under rigorous investigation and has shown promising results.[57-60] Other applications include guiding voice therapy and quantifying outcomes after gender-affirming voice surgery.[61]

Dysphagia

AI models have shown potential to greatly augment efficiency and safety in the evaluation of dysphagia. Once sufficiently robust and well validated, automated aspiration detection from videofluoroscopic swallow studies[62] and flexible endoscopic evaluation of swallowing (FEES)[63] could greatly streamline the diagnostic process and produce standardized evaluation methods. More importantly, the ability to utilize noninvasive high-resolution cervical auscultation for screening and aspiration detection could greatly reduce overall cost and patient exposure to harmful ionizing radiation.[64-67].

Otology

The field of otology has not shied away from exploring opportunities for seamless AI integration to augment everyday practice.

Recently there has been significant success developing models capable of differentiating middle ear pathology from oto-endoscopic images and even images taken from a consumer grade cellular phone otoscope.[68-72] This practical advancement holds potential to democratize ear assessments, reducing unnecessary referrals and making diagnostics more accessible, especially in resource-limited settings. These AI-assisted image classification models have even allowed for the development of shortwave infrared otoscopy approaches, which have shown potential to greatly improve diagnostic accuracy compared to standard visible light otoscopy.[73]

Vestibular pathologies, with their myriad of presentations, require precise differentiation for appropriate management, often resulting in cumbersome office visits that leave the patient with vague uncertainties rather than concrete diagnoses. Deep learning models trained to identify and characterize distinctive exam findings, such as nuanced nystagmus from video recordings,[74] could be quickly integrated into classifier models built to differentiate peripheral from central vestibular pathologies.[75,76] Given the already impressive performance of these preliminary models, once approved for clinical use, implementation could provide rapid feedback to the otolaryngologist in real time, expediting subsequent diagnostic and management decisions.

Owing to intricate anatomy, surgical preparation in otology requires meticulous attention to detail. AI-assisted segmentation of temporal bone scans for facial nerve mapping could greatly aid with this preoperative planning.[77-81] Similar segmentation techniques have been utilized for automated acoustic neuroma identification from radiographical images demonstrating excellent performance metrics for diagnosis, prognostication, and surveillance of these benign tumors.[82-90].

For cochlear implants, models have been developed capable of predicting postoperative outcomes[91-95] and optimization of delivered signals to improve speech intelligibility for their users.[96–103] A source of ongoing debate, these models could lay the foundation for improved eligibility criteria and resulting candidate selection.

Rhinology

The complex world of olfactory disorders, historically reliant on nuanced clinical judgments, is witnessing a surge of AI-driven insights. Results from in-office olfactory function tests have been utilized to identify patterns of olfactory dysfunction associated with specific etiologies such as chronic rhinosinusitis and COVID-19.[104,105] The potential of AI to recognize these etiology-specific patterns offers rhinologists a potentially more refined approach to olfaction-related ailments.

Models informed by noninvasive biomarkers have shown promise in diagnosing eosinophilic chronic rhinosinusitis.[106] Moreover, routinely collected serum lab values have been shown to be effective in risk assessment of nasal polyp recurrence,[107] providing a means to implement proactive management plans for select patients.

An ongoing challenge in rhinology is the objective quantification of disease burden. Currently, there is significant discordance between preoperative symptom severity, radiological findings, and postoperative outcomes. AI, through volumetric assessment techniques, is aiming to ameliorate this discordance via precise quantification of paranasal sinus opacification.[108] Such objectivity, if proven consistently reliable, would be a significant improvement over the reductionist Likert scale approach most commonly utilized. In regards to postoperative outcomes, ensemble learning algorithms have identified specific cytokine profiles derived from mucosal secretions that were independent predictors of decreased symptom burden after endoscopic sinus surgery.[109] Interestingly, similarly generated models from clinico-demographic data alone have shown strong predictive ability for identifying good surgical candidates.[110]

Diagnostic imaging, a cornerstone of rhinology, represents an immense data source that has been leveraged by AI-based models to augment both diagnostics and prognostication. In preliminary studies, these models were capable of differentiating nasal polyps and inverted papillomas using static endoscopic images alone,[111,112] determining malignant transformation of inverted papillomas from preoperative MRI images,[113] and even providing individualized prognostication from histopathologic images of resected polyps.[114]

Likely owing to its multidisciplinary approach, there has been a surge of literature describing the applications of AI in the context of transsphenoidal pituitary resection. These studies have showcased AI's ability to predict both surgical and biochemical outcomes in patients undergoing resection of both functioning and nonfunctioning pituitary adenomas.[115–125] Most exciting are the models capable of identifying patients at risk for intra- and postoperative complications, enabling prediction of cerebrospinal fluid (CSF) leaks, acute diabetes insipidus, and even unplanned 30-day readmission.[126–132]

Sleep medicine

Sleep, though vital, remains a complex physiological process, with dysfunction resulting in a wide range of health consequences. Given the high prevalence of obstructive sleep apnea (OSA), improved efficacy and efficiency of its diagnosis and management could have profound population health and economic implications.

Using data routinely collected in electronic health records, machine learning algorithms were capable of individualized risk stratification for OSA, which could facilitate automated OSA screening expediting diagnosis and subsequent treatment.[133]

AI-driven advances in automated sleep staging from photoplethysmography (PPG) and heart rate variability signals could improve standardization and reduce cost associated with more formal evaluations.[134,135] Moreover, algorithms developed from AI architectures can detect apneic events and even diagnose OSA from PPG signals and even single lead nocturnal electrocardiogram (ECG) recordings.[136–140] These insights from minimal biometric variables reduces need for specialized equipment and, as such, remote monitoring with automated diagnostics from biometric feedback via smart phone applications has already been developed with impressive accuracy.[141]

Offering utility from the perspective of a surgeon, models built from acoustic recordings during sleep were capable of localizing anatomical origin of obstruction, which could greatly aid in targeted operative planning.[142]

Regulatory and ethical considerations

While AI integration brings promises of revolutionized patient care, with it also comes a maze of regulatory, ethical, and reimbursement challenges. As these systems integrate and, in turn, influence healthcare delivery, they will inevitably attract regulatory scrutiny. In the United States, the FDA is largely responsible for this regulatory oversight, and its rigorous criteria for approval broadly focus on the assessment of safety, effectiveness, and generalizability. Input data, algorithmic transparency, and validation methodology are systematically assessed, and performance metrics of the proposed algorithms are benchmarked against existing standard-of-care tools or methods.

Ethically, ensuring informed consent when using AI tools becomes paramount, as does safeguarding the autonomy of clinical judgment and shared decision-making. Liability for the use of AI models should also be considered as both a regulatory and ethical dilemma, as attributing responsibility for clinical decisions derived from AI-generated insights remains unclear.

Challenges and future directions

Despite the promising applications of AI in otolaryngology, several challenges remain, including data quality and availability, model interpretability, and ethical considerations. High-quality, representative datasets are required to develop reliable and generalizable AI models. Furthermore, AI models should be transparent and interpretable to facilitate their adoption by clinicians and acceptance by patients. Ethical considerations, such as data privacy and informed consent, must also be addressed to ensure the responsible implementation of AI in clinical practice.

In addition, AI has the potential to perpetuate and exacerbate existing biases in otolaryngology, particularly if they are trained on unrepresentative or biased datasets. Unfortunately, algorithmic bias is already prevalent in our healthcare system. One algorithm utilized to determine healthcare resource allocation for millions of patients was found to be fraught with racial bias. Under the guidance of this model, black patients were significantly less likely to be identified for supplemental medical resources when compared to white patients with equivalent health needs.[143] Efforts must be taken to ensure that predictions made by AI tools benefit the care of all individuals, including underserved and traditionally marginalized populations.

It is essential to ensure the fairness and equity of AI-driven solutions by employing diverse and representative training datasets, rigorously evaluating algorithm performance across different patient subgroups, and incorporating fairness-aware machine learning techniques.

Conclusion

AI holds great promise for the field, with the potential to transform various aspects of clinical practice, from diagnosis to treatment selection, and prognosis. As technology advances, the integration of AI into clinical practice is expected to become increasingly prevalent, necessitating a thorough understanding of AI principles and methodologies among otolaryngologists. While challenges remain, continued interdisciplinary collaboration, education, and research will drive innovation and ensure the safe, effective, and ethical implementation of AI-driven solutions in otolaryngology.

As AI technology continues to evolve, otolaryngologists must remain proactive in their engagement with AI, embracing the potential benefits while addressing the inherent challenges.

References

1. Narayanan N, Gross AK, Pintens M, Fee C, MacDougall C. Effect of an electronic medical record alert for severe sepsis among ED patients. *Am J Emerg Med*. 2016;34(2): 185−188.

2. McRee L, Thanavaro JL, Moore K, Goldsmith M, Pasvogel A. The impact of an electronic medical record surveillance program on outcomes for patients with sepsis. *Heart Lung*. 2014;43(6):546−549.

3. Fu Q, Chen Y, Li Z, et al. A deep learning algorithm for detection of oral cavity squamous cell carcinoma from photographic images: a retrospective study. *EClinicalMedicine*. 2020;27.

4. Halicek M, Little JV, Wang X, Chen AY, Fei B. Optical biopsy of head and neck cancer using hyperspectral imaging and convolutional neural networks. *J Biomed Opt*. 2019; 24(3), 036007-036007.

5. Coole JB, Brenes D, Mitbander R, et al. Multimodal optical imaging with real-time projection of cancer risk and biopsy guidance maps for early oral cancer diagnosis and treatment. *J Biomed Opt*. 2023;28(1), 016002-016002.

6. Welikala RA, Remagnino P, Lim JH, et al. Automated detection and classification of oral lesions using deep learning for early detection of oral cancer. *IEEE Access*. 2020;8:132677−132693.

7. Bur AM, Holcomb A, Goodwin S, et al. Machine learning to predict occult nodal metastasis in early oral squamous cell carcinoma. *Oral Oncol*. 2019;92:20−25.

8. Farrokhian N, Holcomb AJ, Dimon E, et al. Development and validation of machine learning models for predicting occult nodal metastasis in early-stage oral cavity squamous cell carcinoma. *JAMA Netw Open*. 2022;5(4). e227226-e227226.

9. Oliver JR, Karadaghy OA, Fassas SN, Arambula Z, Bur AM. Machine learning directed sentinel lymph node biopsy in cutaneous head and neck melanoma. *Head Neck*. 2022; 44(4):975−988.

10. Karadaghy OA, Shew M, New J, Bur AM. Development and assessment of a machine learning model to help predict survival among patients with oral squamous cell carcinoma. *JAMA Otolaryngol Head & Neck Surg*. 2019;145(12):1115−1120.

11. Shew M, New J, Bur AM. Machine learning to predict delays in adjuvant radiation following surgery for head and neck cancer. *Otolaryngol Head Neck Surg (Tokyo)*. 2019;160(6):1058−1064.

12. Smith JB, Shew M, Karadaghy OA, et al. Predicting salvage laryngectomy in patients treated with primary nonsurgical therapy for laryngeal squamous cell carcinoma using machine learning. *Head Neck*. 2020;42(9):2330−2339.

13. Keek SA, Wesseling FW, Woodruff HC, et al. A prospectively validated prognostic model for patients with locally advanced squamous cell carcinoma of the head and neck based on radiomics of computed tomography images. *Cancers*. 2021;13(13):3271.

14. Meneghetti AR, Zwanenburg A, Leger S, et al. Definition and validation of a radiomics signature for loco-regional tumour control in patients with locally advanced head and neck squamous cell carcinoma. *Clin Transl Radiat Oncol*. 2021;26:62−70.

15. Wang Y, Lombardo E, Avanzo M, et al. Deep learning based time-to-event analysis with PET, CT and joint PET/CT for head and neck cancer prognosis. *Comput Methods Progr Biomed*. 2022;222:106948.

16. Diamant A, Chatterjee A, Vallières M, Shenouda G, Seuntjens J. Deep learning in head & neck cancer outcome prediction. *Sci Rep*. 2019;9(1):2764.

17. Chen L, Zhou Z, Sher D, et al. Combining many-objective radiomics and 3D convolutional neural network through evidential reasoning to predict lymph node metastasis in head and neck cancer. *Phys Med Biol*. 2019;64(7):075011.

18. Romeo V, Cuocolo R, Ricciardi C, et al. Prediction of tumor grade and nodal status in oropharyngeal and oral cavity squamous-cell carcinoma using a radiomic approach. *Anticancer Res.* 2020;40(1):271−280.

19. Kann BH, Aneja S, Loganadane GV, et al. Pretreatment identification of head and neck cancer nodal metastasis and extranodal extension using deep learning neural networks. *Sci Rep.* 2018;8(1):14036.

20. Ko SY, Lee JH, Yoon JH, et al. Deep convolutional neural network for the diagnosis of thyroid nodules on ultrasound. *Head Neck.* 2019;41(4):885−891.

21. Liu Z, Cao Y, Diao W, Cheng Y, Jia Z, Peng X. Radiomics-based prediction of survival in patients with head and neck squamous cell carcinoma based on pre-and post-treatment 18F-PET/CT. *Aging (Albany NY).* 2020;12(14):14593.

22. Leger S, Zwanenburg A, Pilz K, et al. CT imaging during treatment improves radiomic models for patients with locally advanced head and neck cancer. *Radiother Oncol.* 2019;130:10−17.

23. Tong N, Gou S, Yang S, Ruan D, Sheng K. Fully automatic multi-organ segmentation for head and neck cancer radiotherapy using shape representation model constrained fully convolutional neural networks. *Med Phys.* 2018;45(10):4558−4567.

24. Men K, Chen X, Zhang Y, et al. Deep deconvolutional neural network for target segmentation of nasopharyngeal cancer in planning computed tomography images. *Front Oncol.* 2017;7:315.

25. Outeiral RR, Bos P, Al-Mamgani A, Jasperse B, Simões R, van der Heide UA. Oropharyngeal primary tumor segmentation for radiotherapy planning on magnetic resonance imaging using deep learning. *Physics Imag radiat oncol.* 2021;19:39−44.

26. Van Dijk LV, Van den Bosch L, Aljabar P, et al. Improving automatic delineation for head and neck organs at risk by Deep Learning Contouring. *Radiother Oncol.* 2020; 142:115−123.

27. Van der Veen J, Willems S, Deschuymer S, et al. Benefits of deep learning for delineation of organs at risk in head and neck cancer. *Radiother Oncol.* 2019;138:68−74.

28. Fan J, Wang J, Chen Z, Hu C, Zhang Z, Hu W. Automatic treatment planning based on three-dimensional dose distribution predicted from deep learning technique. *Med Phys.* 2019;46(1):370−381.

29. Lin L, Dou Q, Jin Y-M, et al. Deep learning for automated contouring of primary tumor volumes by MRI for nasopharyngeal carcinoma. *Radiology.* 2019;291(3):677−686.

30. Cardenas CE, McCarroll RE, Court LE, et al. Deep learning algorithm for auto-delineation of high-risk oropharyngeal clinical target volumes with built-in dice similarity coefficient parameter optimization function. *Int J Radiat Oncol Biol Phys.* 2018; 101(2):468−478.

31. Nguyen D, Jia X, Sher D, et al. 3D radiotherapy dose prediction on head and neck cancer patients with a hierarchically densely connected U-net deep learning architecture. *Phys Med Biol.* 2019;64(6):065020.

32. Rhee DJ, Cardenas CE, Elhalawani H, et al. Automatic detection of contouring errors using convolutional neural networks. *Med Phys.* 2019;46(11):5086−5097.

33. Howard FM, Kochanny S, Koshy M, Spiotto M, Pearson AT. Machine learning−guided adjuvant treatment of head and neck cancer. *JAMA Netw Open.* 2020;3(11). e2025881-e2025881.

34. Tseng Y-J, Wang H-Y, Lin T-W, Lu J-J, Hsieh C-H, Liao C-T. Development of a machine learning model for survival risk stratification of patients with advanced oral cancer. *JAMA Netw Open.* 2020;3(8). e2011768-e2011768.

35. Qi M, Li Y, Wu A, et al. Multi-sequence MR image-based synthetic CT generation using a generative adversarial network for head and neck MRI-only radiotherapy. *Med Phys*. 2020;47(4):1880−1894.

36. Dinkla AM, Florkow MC, Maspero M, et al. Dosimetric evaluation of synthetic CT for head and neck radiotherapy generated by a patch-based three-dimensional convolutional neural network. *Med Phys*. 2019;46(9):4095−4104.

37. Zhang Y, Yue N, Su MY, et al. Improving CBCT quality to CT level using deep learning with generative adversarial network. *Med Phys*. 2021;48(6):2816−2826.

38. Maspero M, Houweling AC, Savenije MH, et al. A single neural network for cone-beam computed tomography-based radiotherapy of head-and-neck, lung and breast cancer. *Physics Imag Radiat Oncol*. 2020;14:24−31.

39. Halicek M, Lu G, Little JV, et al. Deep convolutional neural networks for classifying head and neck cancer using hyperspectral imaging. *J Biomed Opt*. 2017;22(6), 060503-060503.

40. Halicek M, Dormer JD, Little JV, et al. Hyperspectral imaging of head and neck squamous cell carcinoma for cancer margin detection in surgical specimens from 102 patients using deep learning. *Cancers*. 2019;11(9):1367.

41. Rodner E, Bocklitz T, von Eggeling F, et al. Fully convolutional networks in multimodal nonlinear microscopy images for automated detection of head and neck carcinoma: pilot study. *Head Neck*. 2019;41(1):116−121.

42. Tang H, Li G, Liu C, et al. Diagnosis of lymph node metastasis in head and neck squamous cell carcinoma using deep learning. *Laryngoscope Investig Otolaryngol*. 2022; 7(1):161−169.

43. Zhang L, Wu Y, Zheng B, et al. Rapid histology of laryngeal squamous cell carcinoma with deep-learning based stimulated Raman scattering microscopy. *Theranostics*. 2019; 9(9):2541.

44. Klein S, Quaas A, Quantius J, et al. Deep learning predicts HPV association in oropharyngeal squamous cell carcinomas and identifies patients with a favorable prognosis using regular H&E stains. *Clin Cancer Res*. 2021;27(4):1131−1138.

45. Das N, Hussain E, Mahanta LB. Automated classification of cells into multiple classes in epithelial tissue of oral squamous cell carcinoma using transfer learning and convolutional neural network. *Neural Network*. 2020;128:47−60.

46. Lee SL, Cabanero M, Hyrcza M, et al. Computer-assisted image analysis of the tumor microenvironment on an oral tongue squamous cell carcinoma tissue microarray. *Clin Transl Radiat Oncol*. 2019;17:32−39.

47. Shaban M, Khurram SA, Fraz MM, et al. A novel digital score for abundance of tumour infiltrating lymphocytes predicts disease free survival in oral squamous cell carcinoma. *Sci Rep*. 2019;9(1):13341.

48. Fang S-H, Tsao Y, Hsiao M-J, et al. Detection of pathological voice using cepstrum vectors: a deep learning approach. *J Voice*. 2019;33(5):634−641.

49. Mathad VC, Scherer N, Chapman K, Liss JM, Berisha V. A deep learning algorithm for objective assessment of hypernasality in children with cleft palate. *IEEE (Inst Electr Electron Eng) Trans Biomed Eng*. 2021;68(10):2986−2996.

50. Fujimura S, Kojima T, Okanoue Y, et al. Classification of voice disorders using a one-dimensional convolutional neural network. *J Voice*. 2022;36(1):15−20.

51. Peng X, Xu H, Liu J, Wang J, He C. Voice disorder classification using convolutional neural network based on deep transfer learning. *Sci Rep*. 2023;13(1):7264.

52. Hu H-C, Chang S-Y, Wang C-H, et al. Deep learning application for vocal fold disease prediction through voice recognition: preliminary development study. *J Med Internet Res.* 2021;23(6):e25247.

53. Powell ME, Rodriguez Cancio M, Young D, et al. Decoding phonation with artificial intelligence (DeP AI): proof of concept. *Laryngoscope Investig Otolaryngol.* 2019; 4(3):328−334.

54. Ren J, Jing X, Wang J, et al. Automatic recognition of laryngoscopic images using a deep-learning technique. *Laryngoscope.* 2020;130(11):E686−E693.

55. Kist AM, Gómez P, Dubrovskiy D, et al. A deep learning enhanced novel software tool for laryngeal dynamics analysis. *J Speech Lang Hear Res.* 2021;64(6):1889−1903.

56. Yousef AM, Deliyski DD, Zacharias SR, de Alarcon A, Orlikoff RF, Naghibolhosseini M. A deep learning approach for quantifying vocal fold dynamics during connected speech using laryngeal high-speed videoendoscopy. *J Speech Lang Hear Res.* 2022;65(6):2098−2113.

57. Tracy JM, Özkanca Y, Atkins DC, Ghomi RH. Investigating voice as a biomarker: deep phenotyping methods for early detection of Parkinson's disease. *J Biomed Inf.* 2020; 104:103362.

58. Ali L, Zhu C, Zhang Z, Liu Y. Automated detection of Parkinson's disease based on multiple types of sustained phonations using linear discriminant analysis and genetically optimized neural network. *IEEE J Transl Eng Health Med.* 2019;7:1−10.

59. Vásquez-Correa JC, Arias-Vergara T, Orozco-Arroyave JR, Eskofier B, Klucken J, Nöth E. Multimodal assessment of Parkinson's disease: a deep learning approach. *IEEE J Biomed Health Inform.* 2018;23(4):1618−1630.

60. Karaman O, Çakın H, Alhudhaif A, Polat K. Robust automated Parkinson disease detection based on voice signals with transfer learning. *Expert Syst Appl.* 2021;178:115013.

61. Bensoussan Y, Pinto J, Crowson M, Walden PR, Rudzicz F, Johns III M. Deep learning for voice gender identification: proof-of-concept for gender-affirming voice care. *Laryngoscope.* 2021;131(5):E1611−E1615.

62. Iida Y, Näppi J, Kitano T, Hironaka T, Katsumata A, Yoshida H. Detection of aspiration from images of a videofluoroscopic swallowing study adopting deep learning. *Oral Radiol.* 2023;39(3):1−10.

63. Weng W, Imaizumi M, Murono S, Zhu X. Expert-level aspiration and penetration detection during flexible endoscopic evaluation of swallowing with artificial intelligence-assisted diagnosis. *Sci Rep.* 2022;12(1):21689.

64. Khalifa Y, Coyle JL, Sejdić E. Non-invasive identification of swallows via deep learning in high resolution cervical auscultation recordings. *Sci Rep.* 2020;10(1):8704.

65. Dudik JM, Coyle JL, El-Jaroudi A, Mao Z-H, Sun M, Sejdić E. Deep learning for classification of normal swallows in adults. *Neurocomputing.* 2018;285:1−9.

66. Mao S, Sabry A, Khalifa Y, Coyle JL, Sejdic E. Estimation of laryngeal closure duration during swallowing without invasive X-rays. *Future Generat Comput Syst.* 2021;115: 610−618.

67. Donohue C, Khalifa Y, Mao S, Perera S, Sejdić E, Coyle JL. Characterizing swallows from people with neurodegenerative diseases using high-resolution cervical auscultation signals and temporal and spatial swallow kinematic measurements. *J Speech Lang Hear Res.* 2021;64(9):3416−3431.

68. Khan MA, Kwon S, Choo J, et al. Automatic detection of tympanic membrane and middle ear infection from oto-endoscopic images via convolutional neural networks. *Neural Network.* 2020;126:384−394.

69. Wu Z, Lin Z, Li L, et al. Deep learning for classification of pediatric otitis media. *Laryngoscope*. 2021;131(7):E2344−E2351.
70. Camalan S, Niazi MKK, Moberly AC, et al. OtoMatch: content-based eardrum image retrieval using deep learning. *PLoS One*. 2020;15(5):e0232776.
71. Zeng X, Jiang Z, Luo W, et al. Efficient and accurate identification of ear diseases using an ensemble deep learning model. *Sci Rep*. 2021;11(1):10839.
72. Cavalcanti TC, Lew HM, Lee K, Lee S-Y, Park MK, Hwang JY. Intelligent smartphone-based multimode imaging otoscope for the mobile diagnosis of otitis media. *Biomed Opt Express*. 2021;12(12):7765−7779.
73. Kashani RG, Młyńczak MC, Zarabanda D, et al. Shortwave infrared otoscopy for diagnosis of middle ear effusions: a machine-learning-based approach. *Sci Rep*. 2021;11(1):12509.
74. Wagle N, Morkos J, Liu J, et al. aEYE: a deep learning system for video nystagmus detection. *Front Neurol*. 2022;13:963968.
75. Ahmadi S-A, Vivar G, Navab N, et al. Modern machine-learning can support diagnostic differentiation of central and peripheral acute vestibular disorders. *J Neurol*. 2020;267:143−152.
76. Tarnutzer A, Weber K. Pattern analysis of peripheral-vestibular deficits with machine learning using hierarchical clustering. *J Neurol Sci*. 2022;434:120159.
77. Wang J, Lv Y, Wang J, et al. Fully automated segmentation in temporal bone CT with neural network: a preliminary assessment study. *BMC Med Imag*. 2021;21:1−11.
78. Hudson TJ, Gare B, Allen DG, Ladak HM, Agrawal SK. Intrinsic measures and shape analysis of the intratemporal facial nerve. *Otol Neurotol*. 2020;41(3):e378−e386.
79. Ke J, Lv Y, Ma F, et al. Deep learning-based approach for the automatic segmentation of adult and pediatric temporal bone computed tomography images. *Quant Imag Med Surg*. 2023;13(3):1577.
80. Li X, Zhu Z, Yin H, Wang Z, Zhuo L, Zhou Y. Labyrinth net: a robust segmentation method for inner ear labyrinth in CT images. *Comput Biol Med*. 2022;146:105630.
81. Jeevakala S, Sreelakshmi C, Ram K, Rangasami R, Sivaprakasam M. Artificial intelligence in detection and segmentation of internal auditory canal and its nerves using deep learning techniques. *Int J Comput Assist Radiol Surg*. 2020;15:1859−1867.
82. Shapey J, Wang G, Dorent R, et al. An artificial intelligence framework for automatic segmentation and volumetry of vestibular schwannomas from contrast-enhanced T1-weighted and high-resolution T2-weighted MRI. *J Neurosurg*. 2019;134(1):171−179.
83. Lee C-c, Lee W-K, Wu C-C, et al. Applying artificial intelligence to longitudinal imaging analysis of vestibular schwannoma following radiosurgery. *Sci Rep*. 2021;11(1):3106.
84. Windisch P, Weber P, Fürweger C, et al. Implementation of model explainability for a basic brain tumor detection using convolutional neural networks on MRI slices. *Neuroradiology*. 2020;62:1515−1518.
85. Abouzari M, Goshtasbi K, Sarna B, et al. Prediction of vestibular schwannoma recurrence using artificial neural network. *Laryngoscope Investig Otolaryngol*. 2020;5(2):278−285.
86. George-Jones NA, Wang K, Wang J, Hunter JB. Automated detection of vestibular schwannoma growth using a two-dimensional U-net convolutional neural network. *Laryngoscope*. 2021;131(2):E619−E624.

87. Neve OM, Chen Y, Tao Q, et al. Fully automated 3D vestibular schwannoma segmentation with and without gadolinium-based contrast material: a multicenter, multivendor study. *Radiology: Artif Intell*. 2022;4(4):e210300.

88. Cass ND, Lindquist NR, Zhu Q, Li H, Oguz I, Tawfik KO. Machine learning for automated calculation of vestibular schwannoma volumes. *Otol Neurotol*. 2022;43(10): 1252—1256.

89. Yu Y, Song G, Zhao Y, Liang J, Liu Q. Prediction of vestibular schwannoma surgical outcome using deep neural network. *World Neurosurgery*. 2023;176:e60—e67.

90. Wang M-y, Jia C-g, Xu H-q, et al. Development and validation of a deep learning predictive model combining clinical and radiomic features for short-term postoperative facial nerve function in acoustic neuroma patients. *Curr Med Sci*. 2023:1—9.

91. Crowson MG, Dixon P, Mahmood R, et al. Predicting postoperative cochlear implant performance using supervised machine learning. *Otol Neurotol*. 2020;41(8): e1013—e1023.

92. Kim H, Kang WS, Park HJ, et al. Cochlear implantation in postlingually deaf adults is time-sensitive towards positive outcome: prediction using advanced machine learning techniques. *Sci Rep*. 2018;8(1):18004.

93. Tan L, Holland SK, Deshpande AK, Chen Y, Choo DI, Lu LJ. A semi-supervised support vector machine model for predicting the language outcomes following cochlear implantation based on pre-implant brain fMRI imaging. *Brain Behav*. 2015;5(12):e00391.

94. Shafieibavani E, Goudey B, Kiral I, et al. Predictive models for cochlear implant outcomes: performance, generalizability, and the impact of cohort size. *Trends Hear*. 2021;25:23312165211066174.

95. Zeitler DM, Buchlak QD, Ramasundara S, Farrokhi F, Esmaili N. Predicting acoustic hearing preservation following cochlear implant surgery using machine learning. *Laryngoscope*. 2023;134(2):926—936.

96. Lai Y-H, Tsao Y, Lu X, et al. Deep learning—based noise reduction approach to improve speech intelligibility for cochlear implant recipients. *Ear Hear*. 2018;39(4):795—809.

97. Grimm R, Pettinato M, Gillis S, Daelemans W. Simulating speech processing with cochlear implants: how does channel interaction affect learning in neural networks? *PLoS One*. 2019;14(2):e0212134.

98. Fischer T, Caversaccio M, Wimmer W. Speech signal enhancement in cocktail party scenarios by deep learning based virtual sensing of head-mounted microphones. *Hear Res*. 2021;408:108294.

99. Kang Y, Zheng N, Meng Q. Deep learning-based speech enhancement with a loss trading off the speech distortion and the noise residue for cochlear implants. *Front Med*. 2021;8:740123.

100. Soleymani R, Selesnick IW, Landsberger DM. SEDA: a tunable Q-factor wavelet-based noise reduction algorithm for multi-talker babble. *Speech Commun*. 2018;96:102—115.

101. Goehring T, Bolner F, Monaghan JJ, Van Dijk B, Zarowski A, Bleeck S. Speech enhancement based on neural networks improves speech intelligibility in noise for cochlear implant users. *Hear Res*. 2017;344:183—194.

102. Bolner F, Goehring T, Monaghan J, Van Dijk B, Wouters J, Bleeck S. *Speech Enhancement Based on Neural Networks Applied to Cochlear Implant Coding Strategies*. IEEE; 2016:6520—6524.

103. Healy EW, Yoho SE, Chen J, Wang Y, Wang D. An algorithm to increase speech intelligibility for hearing-impaired listeners in novel segments of the same noise type. *J Acoust Soc Am*. 2015;138(3):1660—1669.

104. Morse JC, Shilts MH, Ely KA, et al. Patterns of olfactory dysfunction in chronic rhinosinusitis identified by hierarchical cluster analysis and machine learning algorithms. *Int Forum Allergy Rhinol*. 2019;9(3):255−264.

105. Somani SN, Farrokhian N, Macke J, et al. Identifying olfactory phenotypes to differentiate between COVID-19 olfactory dysfunction and sinonasal inflammatory disease. *Otolaryngology-Head Neck Surg (Tokyo)*. 2022;167(5):896−899.

106. Thorwarth RM, Scott DW, Lal D, Marino MJ. Machine learning of biomarkers and clinical observation to predict eosinophilic chronic rhinosinusitis: a pilot study. *Int Forum Allergy Rhinol*. 2021;11(1):8−15.

107. Wang X, Meng Y, Lou H, Wang K, Wang C, Zhang L. Blood eosinophil count combined with asthma history could predict chronic rhinosinusitis with nasal polyp recurrence. *Acta Otolaryngol*. 2021;141(3):279−285.

108. Humphries SM, Centeno JP, Notary AM, et al. Volumetric assessment of paranasal sinus opacification on computed tomography can be automated using a convolutional neural network. *Int Forum Allergy Rhinol*. 2020;10(11):1218−1225.

109. Chowdhury NI, Li P, Chandra RK, Turner JH. Baseline mucus cytokines predict 22-item Sino-Nasal Outcome Test results after endoscopic sinus surgery. *Int Forum Allergy Rhinol*. 2020;10(1):15−22.

110. Nuutinen M, Haukka J, Virkkula P, Torkki P, Toppila-Salmi S. Using machine learning for the personalised prediction of revision endoscopic sinus surgery. *PLoS One*. 2022; 17(4):e0267146.

111. Ay B, Turker C, Emre E, Ay K, Aydin G. Automated classification of nasal polyps in endoscopy video-frames using handcrafted and CNN features. *Comput Biol Med*. 2022;147:105725.

112. Girdler B, Moon H, Bae MR, Ryu SS, Bae J, Yu MS. Feasibility of a deep learning-based algorithm for automated detection and classification of nasal polyps and inverted papillomas on nasal endoscopic images. *Int Forum Allergy Rhinol*. 2021;11(12): 1637−1646.

113. Liu GS, Yang A, Kim D, et al. Deep learning classification of inverted papilloma malignant transformation using 3D convolutional neural networks and magnetic resonance imaging. *Int Forum Allergy Rhinol*. 2022;12(8):1025−1033.

114. Wang K, Ren Y, Ma L, et al. Deep learning-based prediction of treatment prognosis from nasal polyp histology slides. *Int Forum Allergy Rhinol*. 2023;13(5):886−898.

115. Staartjes VE, Serra C, Muscas G, et al. Utility of deep neural networks in predicting gross-total resection after transsphenoidal surgery for pituitary adenoma: a pilot study. *Neurosurg Focus*. 2018;45(5):E12.

116. Agrawal N, Ioachimescu AG. Prognostic factors of biochemical remission after transsphenoidal surgery for acromegaly: a structured review. *Pituitary*. 2020;23:582−594.

117. Zoli M, Staartjes VE, Guaraldi F, et al. Machine learning−based prediction of outcomes of the endoscopic endonasal approach in Cushing disease: is the future coming? *Neurosurg Focus*. 2020;48(6):E5.

118. Zhang W, Sun M, Fan Y, et al. Machine learning in preoperative prediction of postoperative immediate remission of histology-positive Cushing's disease. *Front Endocrinol*. 2021;12:635795.

119. Huber M, Luedi MM, Schubert GA, et al. Machine learning for outcome prediction in first-line surgery of prolactinomas. *Front Endocrinol*. 2022;13:810219.

120. Hollon TC, Parikh A, Pandian B, et al. A machine learning approach to predict early outcomes after pituitary adenoma surgery. *Neurosurg Focus*. 2018;45(5):E8.

121. Liu Y, Liu X, Hong X, et al. Prediction of recurrence after transsphenoidal surgery for Cushing's disease: the use of machine learning algorithms. *Neuroendocrinology*. 2019; 108(3):201−210.

122. Fan Y, Li Y, Li Y, et al. Development and assessment of machine learning algorithms for predicting remission after transsphenoidal surgery among patients with acromegaly. *Endocrine*. 2020;67:412−422.

123. Zanier O, Zoli M, Staartjes VE, et al. Machine learning-based clinical outcome prediction in surgery for acromegaly. *Endocrine*. 2022:1−8.

124. Shu X-j, Chang H, Wang Q, et al. Deep Learning model-based approach for preoperative prediction of Ki67 labeling index status in a noninvasive way using magnetic resonance images: a single-center study. *Clin Neurol Neurosurg*. 2022;219:107301.

125. Chen Y-J, Hsieh H-P, Hung K-C, et al. Deep learning for prediction of progression and recurrence in nonfunctioning pituitary macroadenomas: combination of clinical and MRI features. *Front Oncol*. 2022;12:813806.

126. Voglis S, van Niftrik CH, Staartjes VE, et al. Feasibility of machine learning based predictive modelling of postoperative hyponatremia after pituitary surgery. *Pituitary*. 2020; 23:543−551.

127. Tariciotti L, Fiore G, Carrabba G, et al. A supervised machine learning algorithm predicts intraoperative CSF leak in endoscopic transsphenoidal surgery for pituitary adenomas: model development and prospective validation. *J Neurosurg Sci*. 2021;67(4).

128. Crabb BT, Hamrick F, Campbell JM, et al. Machine learning−based analysis and prediction of unplanned 30-day readmissions after pituitary adenoma resection: a multi-institutional retrospective study with external validation. *Neurosurgery*. 2022;91(2): 263−271.

129. Hou S, Li X, Meng F, Liu S, Wang Z. A machine learning−based prediction of diabetes insipidus in patients undergoing endoscopic transsphenoidal surgery for pituitary adenoma. *World Neurosurgery*. 2023;175.

130. Fuse Y, Takeuchi K, Nishiwaki H, et al. Machine learning models predict delayed hyponatremia post-transsphenoidal surgery using clinically available features. *Pituitary*. 2023;26(2):237−249.

131. Das A. Machine learning driven prediction of cerebrospinal fluid rhinorrhoea following endonasal skull base surgery: a multicentre prospective observational study. *Front Oncol*. 2023;13:1046519.

132. Giordano M, D'Alessandris QG, Chiloiro S, Tariciotti L, Olivi A, Lauretti L. Interpretable machine learning−based prediction of intraoperative cerebrospinal fluid leakage in endoscopic transsphenoidal pituitary surgery: a pilot study. *J Neurol Surg Part B Skull Base*. 2022;83(05):485−495.

133. Ustun B, Westover MB, Rudin C, Bianchi MT. Clinical prediction models for sleep apnea: the importance of medical history over symptoms. *J Clin Sleep Med*. 2016;12(2): 161−168.

134. Uçar MK, Bozkurt MR, Bilgin C, Polat K. Automatic sleep staging in obstructive sleep apnea patients using photoplethysmography, heart rate variability signal and machine learning techniques. *Neural Comput Appl*. 2018;29:1−16.

135. Guillot A, Sauvet F, During EH, Thorey V. Dreem open datasets: multi-scored sleep datasets to compare human and automated sleep staging. *IEEE Trans Neural Syst Rehabil Eng*. 2020;28(9):1955−1965.

136. Khandoker AH, Palaniswami M, Karmakar CK. Support vector machines for automated recognition of obstructive sleep apnea syndrome from ECG recordings. *IEEE Trans Inf Technol Biomed.* 2008;13(1):37−48.

137. Hassan AR, Haque MA. An expert system for automated identification of obstructive sleep apnea from single-lead ECG using random under sampling boosting. *Neurocomputing.* 2017;235:122−130.

138. Khandoker AH, Karmakar CK, Palaniswami M. Automated recognition of patients with obstructive sleep apnoea using wavelet-based features of electrocardiogram recordings. *Comput Biol Med.* 2009;39(1):88−96.

139. Fatimah B, Singh P, Singhal A, Pachori RB. Detection of apnea events from ECG segments using Fourier decomposition method. *Biomed Signal Process Control.* 2020;61: 102005.

140. Uçar MK, Bozkurt MR, Bilgin C, Polat K. Automatic detection of respiratory arrests in OSA patients using PPG and machine learning techniques. *Neural Comput Appl.* 2017; 28:2931−2945.

141. Behar J, Roebuck A, Shahid M, et al. SleepAp: an automated obstructive sleep apnoea screening application for smartphones. *IEEE J Biomed Health Inform.* 2014;19(1): 325−331.

142. Qian K, Janott C, Pandit V, et al. Classification of the excitation location of snore sounds in the upper airway by acoustic multifeature analysis. *IEEE (Inst Electr Electron Eng) Trans Biomed Eng.* 2016;64(8):1731−1741.

143. Obermeyer Z, Powers B, Vogeli C, Mullainathan S. Dissecting racial bias in an algorithm used to manage the health of populations. *Science.* 2019;366(6464):447−453.

The patient perspective on big data and its use in clinical care

Katie Tai, MD [1], **Christopher Babu, BS, Medical Student** [1],
Yeo Eun Kim, BS, Medical Student [1], **Tejas Subramanian, BS, Medical Student** [1],
Anaïs Rameau, MD, MPhil, MS, FACS [2]

[1]*Department of Otolarngology - Head and Neck Surgery, New York Presbyterian - Weill Cornell, New York, NY, United States;* [2]*Sean Parker Institute for the Voice, Weill Cornell Medical College, New York, NY, United States*

As applications of big data and precision medicine aided by artificial intelligence (AI) take hold in clinical medicine, including otolaryngology—head and neck surgery, the patient perspective has become increasingly central to evaluate and incorporate in future research and care. Foremost, medicine serves patients. Understanding patients' concerns and priorities is necessary to build healthy and effective alliances during times of innovative change. This chapter examines the patient perspective on the following topics related to big data: privacy, bias, trust, liability, and engagement.

Privacy

Privacy concerns are a dominant topic when addressing the patient's perspective in precision medicine and AI applications in medicine, as demonstrated in several surveys of the general public.[1-3] This general apprehension should be explored with more scrutiny to better understand the scope of patients' worries about privacy infringement as it relates to big data. The concept of privacy is broad and encompasses several unique but related themes. These include but are not limited to worries about being identified (anonymity), loss of control of how personal information is used (confidentiality/consent), and the safeguarding of information from external threats (security).[4] Each of these themes is substantial, and is at play in big data applications in medicine.

In lay conversation, privacy most commonly refers to the concept of anonymity. Even with concealment of known patient identifiers such as name, birth date, medical record numbers, or social security numbers, there are specific risks involved in

Big Data in Otolaryngology. https://doi.org/10.1016/B978-0-443-10520-3.00004-6

big data and AI research that challenge anonymity. This is particularly true of biometric identifiers. For example, genomic information, even when stripped of identifying labels, is so specific that it may still be used to identify the patient. For example, one study identified people's surnames from profiling short tandem repeats on the Y chromosome and querying public genealogy databases.[5] Within otolaryngology, voice and facial appearance are other examples of biometric identifiers. In the case of voice, from a legal standpoint, only voiceprints or spectrograms are considered identifiers, as voice recognition by earwitnesses declines with time and may not be reliable and objective. It is however not implausible that voice may be used as a unique identifier with further advances in big data and AI. Thus, research groups have noted that simple anonymization and removing common identifiers such as name and medical record numbers is not always sufficient to guarantee nonidentifiability in big data and AI.[6] Additionally, in the United States, each state has its own unique legislation over the handling of biometric identifiers. The Texas attorney general, for instance, recently sued Google for violating consumer protection law by capturing of millions of users' voice and facial data without their consent.[7]

Studies have shown that patients value informed consent in the use of their data for research, but have varying perspectives on what and how much data are used.[8,9] In a study by Lee et al., patients from diverse racial and ethnic groups were asked to provide their perspective on the use of their electronic health record (EHR) data and individual biospecimens in precision medicine research.[8] Many participants across different ethnic groups were content with providing specimens to further research, assuming their data remained confidential and ultimately benefitted others. However, there was considerable concern over the misuse of data to unfairly generate profit or to promote research agendas in more controversial sociopolitical spheres, such as cloning or stem cell research.[8] At a personal level as well, big data have already struggled to address ethical issues regarding unexpected revelations about personal health or family history in direct to consumer genetic testing.[10,11]

Beyond the challenges of anonymity and varying perspectives on informed consent, the protection of patient information presents a constant challenge. Intentional external breaches of security or unintentional data leaks may expose patients' health information. Data are increasingly stored in cloud systems beyond the direct control of health organizations and may be exposed to foreign jurisdictions with different privacy laws and regulations.[12] As large volumes of data are stored with progressively improved quality and specificity, patients' genetic, clinical, or ancestry information may be used to determine their ability to metabolize certain drugs and predict their health risks with high accuracy. This may lead to concern regarding risks of discrimination or even active harm toward those with poor predicted health outcomes or vulnerable genetic profiles. Such concerns about patient data safety are grounded in and exacerbated by recent events, in which public—private partnerships for implementing ML have resulted in privacy breaches. For instance, DeepMind, owned by Alphabet Inc., partnered with the Royal Free London NHS Foundation Trust in 2016 to deploy ML to assist in the management of acute kidney injury.

Google and DeepMind faced class-action lawsuits due to unauthorized use of 1.6 million NHS patients' medical records. They were further criticized for not allocating patients any control over their data use and not engaging in any meaningful discussion regarding data privacy.[13]

Furthermore, patient's perspectives on data privacy are not homogenous. Individuals from racial and ethnic minorities are more concerned about privacy breaches and downstream discrimination,[14] as will be elaborated further in the next section. The type of data at stake may elicit different perspective among patients. For example, participants in focus groups expressed higher level of concern and vulnerability with respect to biospecimens compared to clinical data in the EHR.[8]

Patient perspectives on data privacy as it relates to precision medicine are not necessarily all negative. Some studies have highlighted that patients are willing to sacrifice privacy to contribute to research benefitting future patients.[4] This is especially true for patients who are donating data to research targeting a condition that they or a close family member have experienced.[15,16] Other patients who have participated in direct-to-consumer genetic testing have expressed satisfaction with the safeguards of their privacy and are confident in companies' ability to protect their information—demonstrating that robust data safeguards and communication with patients can ease concerns about privacy breaches.[17] In the public sector, the National Institute of Health (NIH), Food and Drug Administration (FDA), and other government groups have put together task forces and set guidelines for navigating privacy protection in big data and AI.

Despite these advances, many patients still express skepticism that any governance around privacy is effective, and believe that the loss of privacy is an unavoidable part of precision medicine.[4] Understanding and assuaging specific patient concerns regarding privacy through the consent process and beyond is paramount to maintaining patient trust and engagement in big data endeavors.

Demographics and bias within big data
Selecting the patient population

An early and critical process in designing a predictive AI model in clinical and translational medicine involves selecting an initial dataset from which the algorithm learns and develops its subsequent neural networks. Ensuring that the dataset is sufficiently diverse and representative of the intended patient population is essential to its usability and the potential applicability of the predictive model built upon it. Unfortunately, most of data currently available in biorepositories for clinical research are from White Caucasian individuals, which hinders an algorithm's generalizability and inadvertently propagates discriminatory practices.[8,18]

Similar issues arise with sex and gender representation, as recapitulating the known sex and gender bias in healthcare will disproportionately adversely impact women, transgender, and nonbinary individuals in terms of their overall morbidity and mortality.[18–20] For example, a recent study of multiple publicly utilized training datasets for interpreting chest X-ray imaging with AI demonstrated extensive bias against women, as this group was most likely to be incorrectly diagnosed.[21] Interestingly, the proportion of women included in the training set was only marginally smaller than the proportion of men in the cohort, but the algorithm still failed to capture an accurate representation of its target population.[21] Hence, determining an initial training sample is far more complex and nuanced than simply creating a random sample with comparable representation of members of different demographic groups.

Bias within big data and AI

Few studies have evaluated patients' perspectives as contributors of such datasets.[8] There is also a paucity of studies pertaining to how different ethnic and racial groups perceive their participation in big data and AI studies. Patients from racial and ethnic minority groups have reported greater concerns related to AI's bias, especially as it pertains to the risk of misdiagnosis.[14,22,23] Those patients that big data and AI are most likely to inaccurately represent, including women, people of color, nonheterosexual and transgender and nonbinary individuals, also describe concern over the potential of AI to further existing health inequities.[23] Khullar et al. report increased concern over breaches of confidentiality and higher healthcare costs among patients from racial and ethnic minority groups with the introduction of AI technology in healthcare, a trend which was not observed among respondents who identified as White.[14,22]

These patients' suspicion of AI is not unfounded, as there have been several well-documented instances of algorithmic bias within medicine. Seyyed-Kalantari et al. described how a significant portion of underserved populations in medicine, including Medicaid patients, African-American patients, and Hispanic patients, were more likely to be underdiagnosed by AI algorithms designed to identify pathology on routine chest X-ray imaging.[23] Another example frequently discussed in the lay press is the poor accuracy AI machine learning algorithms have in detecting dermatological malignancies in patients with darker skin tones.[24]

AI systems have the potential to utilize deep learning and create iterative networks based on additional datapoints gathered after the initial program has been coded with a training set. In other words, AI continues to grow and adapt to its intended patient population while it gathers data from its new users. Despite this mechanism that helps AI evolve, Hein et al. demonstrated that racial minorities as well as individuals from lower socioeconomic groups are less likely to utilize and engage with digital health tools and thus not contribute new data to algorithm.[25] At first glance, one might surmise that this is because individuals from these groups are intentionally excluded due to human bias. However, the authors also found an association between these marginalized groups and limited digital literacy and access healthcare technology.[25] Thus, bias can be introduced into the system inadvertently through barriers to access, in addition to overt bias. As the AI applies deep learning to further expand its networks, this bias can be amplified and worsen over time.

Bias can also be introduced through sampling errors. AI systems can be built based off of EHR data. However, within a particular EHR, patient data can be represented in vastly different ways. For example, some patients may only present to a healthcare facility with severe presentations of disease and only during acute episodes, causing their "extreme" data to be oversampled. The algorithm will take in the patients' demographic information and clinical data to predict the behavior of future patients. Now if the AI is only aware of these extreme spectrums of disease presentation or only takes into consideration the fragmented episodes of care provided, the system may misinterpret future data from other patients since its frame of reference is skewed.[26] Additionally, fragmentation bias can also be seen among patients from lower socioeconomic status or those patients with poor health literacy that are more often seen in teaching clinics with students and learners. In these settings, data collection may be less reliable and more infrequent, again causing the AI to generate an inaccurate representation of a particular group.[26]

Just as oversampling a particular demographic can skew an AI's perspective, so too can undersampling. For example, certain patient demographics may not be represented at all in a particular region or location, preventing the AI from making accurate predictions if such an individual were to present in the future. Patients who have their care distributed over multiple institutions may also be undersampled, as a predictive model built at any one of these institutions would only receive a partial representation of that individual.[26] The issue of implicit bias among healthcare providers has also long been studied and linked to adverse healthcare outcomes. This bias is especially relevant in big data and AI, since such bias is inherent to the data and the predictive tool cannot detect implicit bias introduced by providers.[14,22,26]

From the evidence available, it is clear that bias exists in AI, but what might be done to help reduce its impact and make this new technology more inclusive to individuals of all backgrounds?

Mitigating the risk of bias

Part of current strategy geared toward mitigating AI's risk of bias involves identifying historically marginalized groups within healthcare that are at risk for being inaccurately represented by the system and making sure they are well represented in a dataset. As such, disabled individuals, geriatric patients, women, and cultural and ethnic minorities have all been identified as groups that require careful attention to prevent implicit and overt bias from affecting a particular algorithm.[27–29] The government and academic and advocacy groups have attempted to bridge the gap between historically disenfranchised patients and inclusion within precision medicine initiatives.

An illustration of the government effort to foster inclusivity in precision medicine is the initiative called, "All of Us" by the NIH.[30] This endeavor is a collaboration with multiple other research centers to create an inclusive precision medicine database that hopes to sample one million individuals from across the United States in order to create a diverse, equitable system that is broadly generalizable and representative of our population. In response to longstanding concern over privacy and data access, the NIH has decided to create an open-access system with confidential, de-identified data for researchers to utilize in their studies. Participants cannot be contacted by researchers and participant data safety is maintained through rigorous security protocols.[30] Similar precision medicine initiatives have been designed by academic centers, such as the University of Michigan's "My PART" study that hopes to mitigate bias in the creation of a diverse biorepository by intentionally enrolling individuals from myriad age, gender, socioeconomic, and racial and ethnic backgrounds.[31] If these attempts at creating a truly diverse, representative biorepository are successful, they would immensely aid the development of AI algorithms that are applicable to our diverse population.

Other means of mitigating bias in existing data samples pertain to the programming structure of an algorithm or predictive model. For instance, as an AI utilizes its learning engine to create its neural networks, explicit commands can be programmed to instruct the system to behave in specific ways when working with its data.[32] The field of cognitive robotics has grown in tandem with AI, seeking to assess and manipulate the ways in which software acquires knowledge and develops understanding.[33] Through further research in this domain, programmers may be better able to equip AI with an ability to filter data in a way that is less prone to generating bias. Furthermore, inclusion of additional protection software, such as adversarial learning and resampling, may help protect against attacks from external entities that attempt to adversely influence AI and prevent AI algorithms from becoming skewed by constantly reassessing its sampling data.[32] As AI continues to evolve, intentional effort will undoubtedly be essential to preventing bias and earning the public's trust.

Trust

Patients' trust in their providers is paramount to the stability and viability of the patient—physician relationship. Patients who trust their provider are more likely to seek care, adhere to prescribed treatment regiments, and feel satisfied with the care they receive, all of which have been shown to result in improved outcomes across medicine.[34–40] In an age of precision medicine, the critical question arises of how big data and AI support a trusting relationship between patients and their providers.

If big data and AI technology are used as part of clinical decision support tools, it is unlikely to dramatically change the existing dynamic of the patient—physician relationship. However, AI already has the potential to exceed the performance of human providers in diagnosis and treatment recommendation, and as the technology strengthens further and is more rooted in clinical practice, the relationship between patients and their physician may shift significantly.[41] There are two areas of concern that may sow distrust in AI-driven technology: (1) accuracy and (2) patient vulnerability.

Accuracy

Medical decision-making is complex, requiring synthesis of the patient's current presentation, past medical history, social history, family history, current medications, allergies, and now genetic history to formulate an effective treatment plan. While big data and AI technology predictive models have proven effective in various aspects of this process, patients express concerns regarding its overall accuracy and the risk of medical errors.[42,43] The algorithms employed are frequently viewed as "black boxes," as current AI technologies are often incapable of explaining the rationale behind the outputs generated.[44,45] Patients and providers alike may not understand how the outputs are generated, feeding an inherent fear of the unknown.[46] Furthermore, a recent large survey demonstrated that while patients have negative perceptions of medical AI, they also have unrealistically positive view of human providers, often believing that human decision-making is superior, contrary to existing evidence.[47] While there are likely a multiplicity of factors contributing to this finding, one may be that when patients perceived greater control over their own health, their trust in physicians increased.[48,49] If decision-making is perceived to be opaque, like the "black box" of AI, there is little sense of control.

Furthermore, as discussed previously, AI algorithms rely on training datasets to build and improve the accuracy of recommendations. An AI model trained with data based on a specific demographic or race will provide recommendations most appropriate for that population and applying it more generally may lead to inaccuracies and bias.[47] In combination, the opacity, novelty, and possible bias of AI stokes distrust in its accuracy.

Patient vulnerability

Patients are a vulnerable population, presenting to the medical system at challenging inflections in their lives. While the practice of medicine is rooted in the trust between physician and providers, patients often feel as if they have little control over their condition and treatment. Especially within marginalized communities, there is already a general mistrust of the medical system following existing healthcare inequalities. The history of egregious events such as the Tuskegee Syphilis Study, or the case of Henrietta Lacks, manifest today as medical provider and research distrust.[50,51] As a result, some patients worry about being taken advantage of by researchers and the technologies they are developing, such as AI. These patients have reservations with how medical institutions, employers, insurance companies, or even the government use personal data and the downstream consequences.[52]

One potential avenue to alleviate distrust is incorporation of machine learning into shared decision-making (SDM). SDM is a core tenant in patient-centered care whereby clinicians and patients make medical decisions together after discussing available evidence. Though oft underutilized, this model has been shown to improve patient satisfaction and outcomes.[53,54] Following, exposure to AI through this model may improve patient trust. However, the use of AI in SDM remains in its infancy. A possible benefit of incorporating AI in SDM is streamlining treatment options and their risks and benefits, allowing physicians more time to build relationships with patients as well as empowering patients to better understand AI recommendations. On the other hand, this system may place the physician in an untenable position as mediator between the AI output and the patient explaining how a recommendation was generated, which is usually not fully understood.[55]

In short, although precision medicine and AI-enabled medical care has the power to revolutionize patient care, there remain several elements that limit patients' trust in its application. Mitigating strategies include incorporating larger datasets with diverse populations over time, and training providers to better understand and communicate the process and recommendations of AI. There is also opportunity for providers to work with medical informatics and data scientists to improve training sets.

Liability and accountability

Even the most judicious practitioner or seamless medical organization has experience with errors in clinical care. These errors may give rise to litigations that aim to hold offending parties accountable and provide a path for patients to obtain reimbursement. While no current litigations currently involve the use of AI in clinical decision-making, with the increasing integration of AI and machine learning in care, concerns have risen about how inaccuracies in the algorithm or other mistakes integrating AI may harm patients.

In the current clinical paradigm, physicians are liable for medical malpractice if they deviate from the standard of care. The NIH and professional groups, most notably in radiology, have begun to discuss reforms and build a standard of care for the implementation of machine learning in clinical care.[56] Having more rigorous regulations for the use of AI is intended to limit the extent of possible harm and provide structure for the still fledgling field. However, such developments such as these in a field as dynamic as precision medicine may also have the unintended consequence of the slowing adoption of AI in medicine and limiting the progression of its potential.

The "black box" problem is a particular acute challenge when it comes to liability, since it may not be possible to provide a trackable reason for why an AI algorithm arrives at the results it provides. The concern here is that this opacifies clinical reasoning and decision-making processes and skirts the standard of care discussion. Furthermore, currently physicians have final decision-making power regarding whether to incorporate AI into clinical care. An interesting area to explore in the future will be consequences for when a physician decides to ignore AI-suggested diagnosis or treatment plans.

Notably, patients have different perspectives than other healthcare stakeholders when considering the accountability of AI in medicine. In a survey comparing views of physicians and the US public, the public is significantly more likely to believe that physicians should be held responsible when an error occurs during care delivered with medical AI. On the other hand, physicians are more likely than the public to believe that vendors and healthcare organizations should be liable for AI-related medical errors.[26]

Data ownership/epistemic inequities

Various private and public organizations are stakeholders in the field of AI in medicine. Healthcare systems and academic centers are aggregators of clinical information and proprietary algorithms for clinical applications and research in AI. In addition, a significant portion of existing technology relating to machine learning and neural networks rests in the hands of large tech corporations.[13] For example, Google, Microsoft, IBM, and Apple are among the many companies competing within the precision medicine sector. Furthermore, information sharing agreements with healthcare organizations can also grant these private organizations access to patient health information. Yet this information originates from patients. As they give external organizations permission to use their data, their unique claim on their own data and the information extracted from it necessarily weakens. As a result, data ownership in the context of AI in medical care has raised questions about epistemic inequities.[57,58]

This element of control and power is something that has been found in focus groups/qualitative studies about AI in medicine.[8] Patients who participate in AI research or precision medicine provide informed consent for the use of their information in research or treatment. However, informed consent often requires significant time investment, and is challenged by both the degree of patient understanding and ability of the consenting party to counsel appropriately about long-term risks without resorting to jargon.[59] The average American patient reads at an eighth-grade reading level, with 20% of Americans reading at a fifth-grade reading level. In one study, 54.8% of patients reported that they did not read the informed consent and in another, only one out of 100 patients spent more than 5 s reading the consent.[60,61] Comprehension of consent is further complicated by the knowledge gap between patients and healthcare professionals. While 85% of patients feel well informed about their treatment after the explanation of the doctor, only 23% of doctors agreed that their patients were well informed.[62] Even among physicians, understanding of AI involvement in medicine varies, with 49% of doctors indicating anxiety or discomfort with using AI in a 2019 survey.[63] Disparities such as these suggest that the current process of consent may not adequately educate patients about the implications of consenting to research care involving big data and AI.

Financial rewards and compensation to patients for contributing their data have also generated controversy as some commentators suggest direct payment could widen inequities by enticing patients to sell their privacy and diminishing the altruism of volunteering for research. For example, in 2015, Amgen offered patients medication at cost in exchange for allowing the company access to personal data.[64] That being said, research participants have demonstrated willingness to give up privacy and control of information in exchange for perceived benefits for future patients.[8] AI has the potential to optimize innovation, improve the efficiency of research/clinical trials, and create beneficial new tools for physicians, consumers, insurers, and regulators.[59] Yet, as detailed in other sections of this chapter, disparity in access and discrimination can limit the benefit for some patient groups. Participants worry about the perpetuation of existing inequities in future iterations of AI that may continue or worsen with more reliance on digital health systems. In addition, despite the promise of AI, current patients are unlikely to experience immediate benefit in care. Conversely, as databases grow more robust and algorithms are refined, biotech and tech companies as well as healthcare organizations thus may stand to benefit from increased funding and power, exacerbating epistemic inequity.

Shift in paradigm: Community engagement

In recent years, the growing field of precision medicine has shifted the focus of biomedical research from local, disease-specific studies to large-scale, population-based research that uses individual biological, environmental, behavioral information to assess genetic and behavioral determinants of health.[65] To address the issues of community trust, participant engagement, and ethical concerns that have been associated with both AI and precision medicine, researchers have sought ways to empower participants as equal stakeholders.

Most notably, many studies have promoted participant autonomy through robust informed consent processes that ensure voluntary participation and improved understanding via considerations for health literacy.[47] Other initiatives, such as the enhancement of institutional trustworthiness, dissemination of appropriate resources, and establishment of partnered workgroups comprised both local community and academic teams, have aimed to increase transparency and participant engagement.[66] Despite all these efforts, study design is still mostly being driven by academic or industry research groups, with little to no participant input. This imbalance in power contributes to the slow acceptance of AI and precision medicine research in the community and exacerbates the already existing disparities in big data.

As a solution to this, many academic institutions have turned to *community-engaged research*. Community-engaged research focuses on facilitating cooperation and engagement between community members, academics, and healthcare providers. This involves creating an environment conducive to sharing the underlying challenges and social concerns that are difficult to uncover in traditional technology-oriented and researcher-centered approaches.[67] To achieve this, it is crucial to cultivate long-term, trusting relationships with participants, especially among underresourced communities and underrepresented groups with historical concerns about biomedical research. Navigating cultural, religious, and language barriers can elucidate the specific risks and benefits for different communities, which will ultimately help integrate patient values and expectations into research design and governance structures.[47]

Perhaps one of the greatest barriers to achieving community engagement is the failure of big data research to provide information that is easily accessible and understandable by the public. Therefore, it is only natural that more and more clinical researchers are adopting and partnering with patient-centered, patient-driven efforts for developing platforms for enrolling and monitoring their participation. For example, Recurrent Respiratory Papillomatosis Foundation is a patient-driven organization that has partnered with CoRDS, a centralized international patient registry that patients can enroll in for free. This has helped patients and families take ownership of their medical condition and connected them to advocacy groups and leading researchers in the field.[68]

In addition to patient registries, advocacy groups and mobile health apps have played an integral role in further closing the information gap between patients and healthcare providers.[69] Many novel precision medicine approaches are utilizing technologies, such as Internet of Things, smart devices, and voice-recognition systems, to collect new types of data more frequently. Information gathered from individual users will not only help providers deliver more personalized healthcare to individual patients but also will add to the ever-growing collection of big data. However, these new modes of data collection are not without fail. Although empowering for those who have access, this trend places older and less affluent individuals with less digital literacy at a significant disadvantage. The support of family and advocacy groups and the development of user-friendly interfaces are crucial for transmitting information to and the fair representation of such underrepresented groups.[69] Generating an unbiased database that is representative of the population will ultimately help increase the accuracy and precision of AI-driven models.

Finally, advancements in AI and ML have provided novel ways to enhance patient engagement. A recent study used ML and natural language processing (NLP) to extract messages from social media as real-time assessments of patients' quality of life. Such patient-generated data provide insight into patient concerns and unmet needs that can then be addressed by public health experts, healthcare professionals, and pharmaceutical companies.[70] This can help facilitate real-time, streamlined communication between patients and providers, which may lead to improved patient experience and better healthcare outcomes. Remote patient monitoring (RPM) is a novel concept that also harnesses the power of AI. This allows patient data to be gathered outside of traditional healthcare settings, enabling physicians to monitor and provide care to patients even after their discharge. Notably, UCI Health, with its partner Biofourmis, recently announced the launch of a virtual care platform for RPM and its hospital-at-home initiative, aimed to optimize treatment, predict outcomes, and improve patient engagement with treatment.[71]

It is without a doubt that recent advancements in precision medicine require researchers to respect and involve participants as equal stakeholders in a shared enterprise. AI and ML have and will continue to help increase community engagement allowing for improved communication and better healthcare delivery.

References

1. Hull SC, Sharp RR, Botkin JR, et al. Patients' views on identifiability of samples and informed consent for genetic research. *Am J Bioeth.* 2008;8(10):62–70.
2. Garrison NA, Sathe NA, Antommaria AH, et al. A systematic literature review of individuals' perspectives on broad consent and data sharing in the United States. *Genet Med.* 2016;18(7):663–671.
3. Sanderson SC, Brothers KB, Mercaldo ND, et al. Public attitudes toward consent and data sharing in biobank research: a large multi-site experimental survey in the US. *Am J Hum Genet.* 2017;100(3):414–427.
4. Clayton EW, Halverson CM, Sathe NA, Malin BA. A systematic literature review of individuals' perspectives on privacy and genetic information in the United States. *PLoS One.* 2018;13(10):e0204417.
5. Gymrek M, McGuire AL, Golan D, Halperin E, Erlich Y. Identifying personal genomes by surname inference. *Science.* 2013;339(6117):321–324.
6. Azencott CA. Machine learning and genomics: precision medicine versus patient privacy. *Philos Trans A Math Phys Eng Sci.* 2018;376(2128).
7. Bushard B. *Texas AG Sues Google for Allegedly Capturing Face and Voice Data Without Consent*; 2022. Available from: forbes.com/sites/brianbushard/2022/10/20/amazon-faces-1-billion-uk-suit-latest-alleged-antitrust-violation-against-the-company-1/?sh=400 649375bc8.
8. Lee SS, Cho MK, Kraft SA, et al. I don't want to be Henrietta Lacks": diverse patient perspectives on donating biospecimens for precision medicine research. *Genet Med.* 2019;21(1):107–113.
9. Fosch-Villaronga E, Drukarch H, Khanna P, Verhoef T, Custers B. Accounting for diversity in AI for medicine. *Comput Law Secur Rev.* 2022;47.
10. What Unexpected Things Might I Learn From 23andMe?. Available from: What Unexpected Things Might I Learn From 23andMe?.
11. Brodwin E. After you spit into a tube for a DNA test like 23andMe, experts say you shouldn't assume your data will stay private forever. *Business Insider*; 2019 [Available from: https://www.businessinsider.com/privacy-security-risks-genetic-testing-23andme-ancestry-dna-2019-2.
12. Malin BA, Emam KE, O'Keefe CM. Biomedical data privacy: problems, perspectives, and recent advances. *J Am Med Inform Assoc.* 2013;20(1):2–6.
13. Murdoch B. Privacy and artificial intelligence: challenges for protecting health information in a new era. *BMC Med Ethics.* 2021;22(1):122.
14. Khullar D, Casalino LP, Qian Y, Lu Y, Krumholz HM, Aneja S. Perspectives of patients about artificial intelligence in health care. *JAMA Netw Open.* 2022;5(5):e2210309.
15. Nagaraj CB, Rothwell E, Hart K, Latimer S, Schiffman JD, Botkin JR. Attitudes of parents of children with serious health conditions regarding residual bloodspot use. *Public Health Genom.* 2014;17(3):141–148.

16. Kaphingst KA, Janoff JM, Harris LN, Emmons KM. Views of female breast cancer patients who donated biologic samples regarding storage and use of samples for genetic research. *Clin Genet*. 2006;69(5):393—398.

17. Bollinger JM, Green RC, Kaufman D. Attitudes about regulation among direct-to-consumer genetic testing customers. *Genet Test Mol Biomarkers*. 2013;17(5):424—428.

18. Muñoz DC, Sant C, Becedas RR, Fat DM. *Dangers of gender bias in CRVS and cause of death data: the path to health inequality*. 2022:1—24.

19. Carnevale A, Tangari EA, Iannone A, Sartini E. Will big data and personalized medicine do the gender dimension justice? *AI Soc*. 2021;38.

20. Seyyed-Kalantari L, Liu G, McDermott M, Chen IY, Ghassemi M. CheXclusion: fairness gaps in deep chest X-ray classifiers. *Pac Symp Biocomput*. 2021;26:232—243.

21. Hein AE, Vrijens B, Hiligsmann M. A digital innovation for the personalized management of adherence: analysis of strengths, weaknesses, opportunities, and threats. *Front Med Technol*. 2020;2.

22. Norori N, Hu Q, Aellen FM, Faraci FD, Tzovara A. Addressing bias in big data and AI for health care: a call for open science. *Patterns (N Y)*. 2021;2:100347.

23. Seyyed-Kalantari L, Zhang H, McDermott MBA, Chen IY, Ghassemi M. Underdiagnosis bias of artificial intelligence algorithms applied to chest radiographs in under-served patient populations. *Nat Med*. 2021;27(12):2176—2182.

24. Lashbrook A. AI-driven dermatology could leave dark-skinned patients behind. *Atlantic*. Aug 16, 2018.

25. Gianfrancesco MA, Tamang S, Yazdany J, Schmajuk G. Potential biases in machine learning algorithms using electronic health record data. *JAMA Intern Med*. 2018;178:1544—1547.

26. Khullar D, Casalino LP, Qian Y, Lu Y, Chang E, Aneja S. Public vs physician views of liability for artificial intelligence in health care. *J Am Med Inf Assoc : JAMIA*. 2021;28:1574—1577.

27. Chu CH, Nyrup R, Leslie K, et al. Digital ageism: challenges and opportunities in artificial intelligence for older adults. *Gerontol*. 2022;62(7):947—955.

28. Gupta M, Parra CM, Dennehy D. Questioning racial and gender bias in AI-based recommendations: do espoused national cultural values matter? *Inf Syst Front : A J Res Innovat*. 2021:1—17. Advance online publication.

29. Lillywhite A, Wolbring G. Coverage of ethics within the artificial intelligence and machine learning academic literature: the case of disabled people. *Assist Technol : Off J RESNA*. 2021;33:129—135.

30. All of US Research Program. National Institutes of Health (NIH); Available from: https://allofus.nih.gov/.

31. My Part. University of Michigan Precision Health; Available from: https://precisionhealth.umich.edu/our-research/my-part/.

32. Cirillo D, Catuara-Solarz S, Morey C, et al. Sex and gender differences and biases in artificial intelligence for biomedicine and healthcare. *NPJ Digit Med*. 2020;3:81.

33. Ognibene D, Foulsham T, Marchegiani L, Farinella GM. Active vision and perception in human-robot collaboration. *Front Neurorob*. 2022;16.

34. Schoenthaler A, Montague E, Baier Manwell L, Brown R, Schwartz MD, Linzer M. Patient-physician racial/ethnic concordance and blood pressure control: the role of trust and medication adherence. *Ethn Health*. 2014;19(5):565—578.

35. Piette JD, Heisler M, Krein S, Kerr EA. The role of patient-physician trust in moderating medication nonadherence due to cost pressures. *Arch Intern Med.* 2005;165(15): 1749–1755.

36. Nguyen GC, LaVeist TA, Harris ML, Datta LW, Bayless TM, Brant SR. Patient trust-in-physician and race are predictors of adherence to medical management in inflammatory bowel disease. *Inflamm Bowel Dis.* 2009;15(8):1233–1239.

37. Hall MA, Dugan E, Zheng B, Mishra AK. Trust in physicians and medical institutions: what is it, can it be measured, and does it matter? *Milbank Q.* 2001;79(4):613–639, v.

38. Berry LL, Parish JT, Janakiraman R, et al. Patients' commitment to their primary physician and why it matters. *Ann Fam Med.* 2008;6(1):6–13.

39. Haskard KB, DiMatteo MR, Heritage J. Affective and instrumental communication in primary care interactions: predicting the satisfaction of nursing staff and patients. *Health Commun.* 2009;24(1):21–32.

40. Lee YY, Lin JL. The effects of trust in physician on self-efficacy, adherence and diabetes outcomes. *Soc Sci Med.* 2009;68(6):1060–1068.

41. Davenport T, Kalakota R. The potential for artificial intelligence in healthcare. *Future Healthc J.* 2019;6(2):94–98.

42. Esmaeilzadeh P. Use of AI-based tools for healthcare purposes: a survey study from consumers' perspectives. *BMC Med Inform Decis Mak.* 2020;20(1):170.

43. Topol EJ. High-performance medicine: the convergence of human and artificial intelligence. *Nat Med.* 2019;25(1):44–56.

44. Wischmeyer T. Artificial intelligence and transparency: Opening the black box. *Regulat Artificial Intelligence.* 2020;75.

45. Price 2nd WN, Gerke S, Cohen IG. How much can potential jurors tell us about liability for medical artificial intelligence? *J Nucl Med.* 2021;62(1):15–16.

46. Wadden JJ. Defining the undefinable: the black box problem in healthcare artificial intelligence. *J Med Ethics.* 2021;48.

47. Kraft SA, Cho MK, Gillespie K, et al. Beyond consent: building trusting relationships with diverse populations in precision medicine research. *Am J Bioeth.* 2018;18(4):3–20.

48. Cadario R, Longoni C, Morewedge CK. Understanding, explaining, and utilizing medical artificial intelligence. *Nat Hum Behav.* 2021;5(12):1636–1642.

49. Gabay G. Perceived control over health, communication and patient-physician trust. *Patient Educ Couns.* 2015. https://doi.org/10.1016/j.pec.2015.06.019.

50. Rajakumar K, Thomas SB, Musa D, Almario D, Garza MA. Racial differences in parents' distrust of medicine and research. *Arch Pediatr Adolesc Med.* 2009;163(2): 108–114.

51. Gamble VN. A legacy of distrust: African Americans and medical research. *Am J Prev Med.* 1993;9(6 Suppl):35–38.

52. Bari L, O'Neill DP. Rethinking patient data privacy in the era of digital health. *Health Aff Forefront.* 2019.

53. Shay LA, Lafata JE. Where is the evidence? A systematic review of shared decision making and patient outcomes. *Med Decis Making.* 2015;35(1):114–131.

54. Hughes TM, Merath K, Chen Q, et al. Association of shared decision-making on patient-reported health outcomes and healthcare utilization. *Am J Surg.* 2018;216(1):7–12.

55. Abbasgholizadeh Rahimi S, Cwintal M, Huang Y, et al. Application of artificial intelligence in shared decision making: scoping review. *JMIR Med Inform.* 2022;10(8):e36199.

56. Maliha G, Gerke S, Cohen IG, Parikh RB. Artificial intelligence and liability in medicine: balancing safety and innovation. *Milbank Q.* 2021;99(3):629–647.

57. Leonelli S. What difference does quantity make? on the epistemology of big data in biology. *Big Data Soc.* 2014;1(1).

58. Leonelli S. The challenges of big data biology. *Elife.* 2019;8.

59. Erdmann A, Rehmann-Sutter C, Bozzaro C. Patients' and professionals' views related to ethical issues in precision medicine: a mixed research synthesis. *BMC Med Ethics.* 2021; 22(1):116.

60. Andrew Coombes OL. Investigations of doctors by general medical council. *BMJ;* 2000. Available from: https://www.bmj.com/rapid-response/2011/10/28/do-patients-read-consent-forms.

61. Ozhan MO, Suzer MA, Comak I, et al. Do the patients read the informed consent? *Balkan Med J.* 2014;31(2):132−136.

62. Ciardiello F, Adams R, Tabernero J, et al. Awareness, understanding, and adoption of precision medicine to deliver personalized treatment for patients with cancer: a multinational survey comparison of physicians and patients. *Oncol.* 2016;21(3):292−300.

63. Frellick M. *AI Use in Healthcare Increasing Slowly Worldwide.* MedScape; 2019. Available from: https://www.medscape.com/viewarticle/912629?icd=login_success_gg_match_norm.

64. Prainsack B, Forgo N. Why paying individual people for their health data is a bad idea. *Nat Med.* 2022;28(10):1989−1991.

65. Sahu M, Gupta R, Ambasta RK, Kumar P. Artificial intelligence and machine learning in precision medicine: a paradigm shift in big data analysis. *Prog Mol Biol Transl Sci.* 2022; 190(1):57−100.

66. Jones L, Wells K, Lin HJ, et al. Community partnership in precision medicine: themes from a community engagement conference. *Ethn Dis.* 2018;28(Suppl 2):503−510.

67. Hsu YC, Huang T, Verma H, Mauri A, Nourbakhsh I, Bozzon A. Empowering local communities using artificial intelligence. *Patterns (N Y).* 2022;3(3):100449.

68. Foundation RRP. Global RRPF/CoRDS RRP Patient Registry. Available from: https://rrpf.org/cords-global-patient-registry/.

69. MacMartin-Moglia K, Mahler M. Chapter 12 - precision medicine from the patient's perspective: more opportunities and increasing responsibilities. In: Mahler M, ed. *Precision Medicine and Artificial Intelligence.* Academic Press; 2021:267−277.

70. Renner S, Marty T, Khadhar M, et al. A new method to extract health-related quality of life data from social media testimonies: algorithm development and validation. *J Med Internet Res.* 2022;24(1):e31528.

71. McNemar E. *UCI Health Aims to Improve Remote Patient Monitoring via AI Partnership.* 2022.

Index

9780443105203